THE ROYAL WAY

GROW YOUR PRACTICE

VIDISHA CHAMRIA

BlueRoseONE.com
Stories Matter
NewDelhi • London

BLUEROSE PUBLISHERS
India | U.K.

BlueRose ONE.com
Stories Matter
NewDelhi • London

For permissions requests or inquiries regarding this publication, please contact:

BLUEROSE PUBLISHERS
www.BlueRoseONE.com
info@bluerosepublishers.com
+91 8882 898 898
+4407342408967

ISBN: 978-93-6261-202-1

Cover design: Tahira
Typesetting: Tanya Raj Upadhyay

First Edition: December 2024

Foreword

In life's grand tapestry, photographs often serve as memorials, particularly poignant after one's passing. Criticism is a burden borne by the living, while memories immortalize the departed. This biography transcends snapshots, capturing a man's extraordinary journey.

Welcome to 'Grow Your Practice,' a tribute to an extraordinary individual whose relentless dedication and profound wisdom have inspired countless others. This book delves into the remarkable journey of Dr. Arun Chamria, tracing his evolution from a young boy to a loving son, devoted father, cherished grandfather, respected doctor, loyal husband, and above all, an exceptional human being.

Swami Chinmayananda advised seeing oneself in Krishna's role while reading the Bhagavad Gita, offering insights into handling life's challenges. Similarly, as you read, reflect on how you might have navigated Dr Arun's experiences. Was his approach commendable or merely adequate? This introspection fosters personal growth and enhances societal contribution.

Dr Arun's story begins with dentistry and culminates with his family, reflecting his unwavering commitment. Every day, he lived and breathed dentistry. This book is for those intrigued by a young man's life and those seeking a fresh perspective on dentistry. Join this journey with an open heart, letting Arun's story inspire reflection, growth, and a new outlook on life.

Table of Contents

Visionary Behind 'The Royal Ritual': Dr. Arun Chamria

Growing up in the small village of Fatehpur in Rajasthan, as a young boy like any other, Arun faced numerous challenges. Diagnosed with liver disease, his childhood was marked by a highly restrictive diet. And with the simple family background, the spendings were also regulated. Young Arun, however, would sneak sweets in exchange for homework help, showing an early knack for negotiation and resilience.

At the time of Arun's birth, his father was studying at BITS, Pilani one of the most prestigious engineering colleges in India. Arun and his mother, and his sister, grew up in Fatehpur, Rajasthan along with extended family. During his childhood, he recalls their move to Mumbai to join his father. With three growing children and a wife, his father's income was just enough to afford the basic necessities of life.

The family belonged to working class. They had money, but a lavish lifestyle was beyond their reach. Responsibilities, relationships, and rules shaped their lives. A common aspect of their everyday life was that their favourite fruit was the banana, simply because everything else was considered to be a luxury.

Arun Chamria's journey into dentistry was more than a career choice; it was a calling born out of trials and tribulations. Despite these hardships, Arun excelled academically and remained determined to pursue his dreams. Living in a household of about 25 people with extended families, he learned the values of community and empathy, early.

A Turn of Fate: Dr. Arun pursued Dentistry

Arun aspired to become a doctor and worked tirelessly to get into an MBBS program. However, just before his crucial entrance exams, a close relative passed away, deeply affecting him and distracting him from his studies. That year, a significant reduction in MBBS seats meant that despite excellent marks, Arun narrowly missed securing a spot.

Initially, Arun viewed dentistry as a compromise. I believe this speaks for a lot of other fields too, but it's about doing what's best in our hands. He soon discovered a profound passion for the field. His precision and empathy made him an exceptional dentist, turning what seemed like a setback into a fulfilling career dedicated to patient care.

Early Life Lessons from Cricket

Arun was an ardent cricket fan, so passionate that if the film '83 had been released in his presence, he could have narrated the script in advance. He loved playing cricket, but his mother was always worried about his studies. Every Sunday, Arun would head out with his friends at 7:30 a.m. and return home just before sunset. To sway his mother, he would charm her with a few lines and hugs before vanishing to play.

His two sisters often helped convince their mother, and Arun would barter chocolates with them for their assistance.

Arun's love for cricket was another significant part of his childhood. Due to his health conditions, he often played with much older boys, teaching him valuable lessons in leadership, diplomacy, and resilience. These early experiences helped him develop strategies to negotiate and earn respect, skills that proved crucial in his professional life.

Cricket in India has always been more than a sport, it's been an emotion. Playing cricket with older boys wasn't just a game; it was a classroom for life lessons. Arun had to navigate complex social dynamics, learn to stand his ground and prove his worth through performance and conduct. These skills translated seamlessly into his professional life, where leadership, negotiation, and resilience are essential. How cricket is a game of multiple players at the field, even Dentistry in healthcare requires multiple players and managing them requires great leadership.

Big Game: Lesson in Persuasion & Management

Arun had the privilege of attending convent school, which was a rare opportunity for anybody in those days. Despite financial concerns and social stigma, his parents decided to enrol his two younger sisters in the same convent school. Meeting the expenses was a challenge, but his father believed in providing equal educational opportunities to both genders, emphasizing that boys and girls should have access to the best schooling.

Arun's younger sister struggled with Mathematics, so their father tasked Arun with teaching her. He often reminded Arun, "You are an elder brother and it is your duty to help your siblings; otherwise, your education is of no use." Arun's father believed that while free knowledge might not always be respected, imparting life lessons would always pay off in some way.

At 17, Arun and his friends organized a big game fair in their community. Securing necessary permissions required Arun to demonstrate remarkable leadership and persuasion skills. He convinced local authorities and even persuaded the local MLA to attend as the chief guest. The fair was a success, teaching Arun the importance of initiative, strategic planning, and financial management.

This event wasn't just a fair; it was a milestone in Arun's life. Convincing the local authorities and the MLA showcased his ability to communicate effectively and present a compelling case. The fair's success demonstrated his capacity to plan, execute, and manage resources efficiently, laying the groundwork for his future endeavours.

Unexpected Offer: Special Executive Magistrate

At a very early age, Arun got multiple opportunities and excelled in making use of them. When he turned 21, he was unexpectedly offered the prestigious post of Special Executive Magistrate. Awed by the attention and responsibilities, Arun was eager to accept. However, his father, a disciplined and dynamic man, advised against it, believing it would divert Arun's focus from his medical ambitions. This taught Arun the importance of prioritizing his goals and maintaining discipline.

Arun's father played a crucial role in shaping his son’s priorities, teaching him the value of commitment and long-term planning. This lesson proved invaluable as Arun navigated the challenges and opportunities in his professional journey.

One such instance, Baluram Halwai, a Brahmin who cooked for Arun's family and whose Sattvic food was highly cherished, faced his own challenges. When his daughter’s marriage was fixed, he lacked sufficient savings and needed financial support. Arun's father, showing his compassionate nature, decided to help. The entire family attended the wedding and enjoyed the events. When the groom’s family requested ice cream for dessert, Baluram, feeling helpless, explained he could not afford it. Demonstrating their generosity, Arun’s father spent Rs 2500 on ice creams, a significant amount in the 1980s.

Despite their own financial challenges, Arun’s father gathered the family that evening and said, "If God has made us capable, then why take a step back?" This moment, much like the decision regarding the Special Executive Magistrate post, underscored the importance of compassion, prioritizing family, and maintaining discipline in life.

Lessons in Humility and Graciousness

At the age of 23, in his final year of dental school, Arun ran for elections for the General Secretary of the student body but lost. His father advised him to personally congratulate the winner, teaching him a valuable lesson in humility and graciousness. This act earned him respect and a lasting friendship with his opponent. This experience was a turning point in Arun's life, teaching him to accept defeat gracefully and build relationships even in the face of competition. These qualities of humility and collaboration became cornerstones of his professional and personal life, helping him build a successful practice and lasting connections.

Arun also played a significant role in the Leo Club of Malad East, where he served as president for three years. The club held board meetings once a month on Friday nights at restaurants, often running late into the night. Arun's younger sibling also aspired to hold a post in the club, specifically as a director. Recognizing this desire, Arun, who was always overprotective, created a new post of Educational Director. He ensured that all meetings related to educational affairs were held on Sundays at their home, supporting his sibling's involvement while maintaining a balance between responsibility and family support.

Through both experiences, Arun demonstrated the importance of humility in victory and defeat, and the value of supporting and uplifting others. These principles guided him throughout his life, shaping his approach to leadership and personal relationships.

Innovative Thinking: Lessons in Business Principle

Despite losing the election, Arun became the Chief Editor of the college magazine, where he demonstrated his innovative spirit by implementing the principle of supply and demand. He limited advertisements to premium slots, generating significant revenue and transforming the struggling publication into a profitable venture. This experience laid the groundwork for Arun's future business endeavours, including the creation of the "Magic" magazine for the Malad Medical Association. His approach of creating scarcity and focusing on quality over quantity showcased his entrepreneurial mindset, teaching him valuable business principles that he later applied in his dental practice.

Arun's innovative spirit wasn't limited to his professional life. On Rakhi festival, despite financial constraints, he always wanted to get something special for his sisters out of his own money. He would save diligently, often skipping his favourite vada pav, to give them meaningful gifts. One memorable occasion was when he saved for an entire month to buy green-stoned oval-shaped earrings and a locket for his sisters, making it the best gift ever. These small yet significant acts of love and innovation in his personal life highlighted his dedication and resourcefulness, principles that he carried into every aspect of his life.

Through these experiences, Arun exemplified innovation as a core principle, both in his professional achievements and personal gestures. His ability to think creatively and prioritize quality and meaning over mere quantity was a defining trait that influenced his successful career and cherished family relationships.

Entering into Dentistry: Peoples Perspective

Looking at Arun's life, he was surrounded by people and relations imparting good virtues and helping him become better each day. It's this ambience that helps one unfold the goodness which is inside each one of us. Let us now delve into his better half, the dental practice.

In the late 80s, when someone mentioned dentistry, it often evoked two common responses: "Find a dentist near your home because you'll need multiple visits," or, "Are you visiting the dentist to get your teeth removed?" Dentistry was primarily associated with extraction rather than prevention or regular care. This perception often demotivated those pursuing a career in dentistry, as the field was seen more as a necessity for dealing with problems than for maintaining oral health. Prevention and routine dental care were not as emphasized, shaping a rather limited view of the profession at that time.

In the early years of Arun's practice, one very close acquaintance of Dr. Arun visited him for a consultation. The acquaintance's dismissive outlook towards dentistry, seeing it merely as a profession for extracting teeth at Rs 15 and giving dentures for Rs 15, was hurtful. This moment became a turning point for Dr. Chamria. He decided then to change the public's perception of dentistry, which indeed triggered the birth to *The Royal Ritual.*

Challenging norms of Practice: The Royal Ritual

Dr. Chamria challenged the routine dental practice at every step. He observed, learned, and implemented innovative ideas that set his practice apart. He elevated the patient care experience by serving water in silverware, hiring a dedicated interior designer to create an aesthetically pleasing clinic, having waiting rooms for patients, and traveling across the globe to learn about new technologies. While these practices might seem normal today, they were ground-breaking in the 1980s.

Dr. Chamria realized early on that dentistry and technology go hand in hand. He adopted the latest technology in his practice from the very beginning, a norm that holds true even today. His relentless pursuit of excellence led him to learn from the best in the world and bring innovations like Same-Day Dentistry to India. He educated himself and his team, continually pushing the boundaries of what was possible in dental care.

Inspired by a talk by Dr. Blatchford in the early 2000s, Dr. Chamria adopted a patient-centric approach to dentistry. Dr. Blatchford emphasized viewing dentistry from the patient's perspective and considering the competition not as other dentists but as other industries like luxury hotels and airlines. This mindset led Dr. Chamria to eliminate waiting times, ensuring no queues and providing dedicated patient waiting rooms.

Dr. Chamria also recognized that extended timelines for dental treatments often resulted in an incomplete care. To counter this, he introduced a policy of full payment in advance, which reinforced the commitment to deliver on promises. Additionally, he implemented a system of zero fees for routine visits. This approach was inspired by an encounter with a Gujarati diamond merchant who sought treatment elsewhere after experiencing issues with his prosthesis. The patient's eventual relief from another dentist, Dr. Mirza (Dr. Chamria's former mentor), taught Dr.

Chamria the crucial importance of maintaining a balanced occlusion.

This realization led to a significant change in his practice. Dr. Chamria developed a policy where any patient experiencing trouble with treatment could return without follow-up fees. This approach ensured that patients would seek solutions directly from him, allowing him to address issues comprehensively. This policy benefited patients by alleviating cost burdens and motivated the clinic to find long-term solutions.

Reflection: Dr Arun's Passion & Dedication

Dr. Chamria's journey is a testament to passion, dedication, and compassionate care. Here are three cases that profoundly influenced his approach:

- **Holistic Patient Care:** A woman with severe burning during eating found relief after Dr. Chamria diagnosed her low haemoglobin levels. This experience highlighted the importance of holistic care. The patient's relief and subsequent health improvement underscored the importance of looking beyond the immediate symptoms and considering the overall well-being of the patient. Dr. Chamria's holistic approach ensured comprehensive care, setting a precedent for his practice.
- **Perseverance:** A patient from the USA, previously denied treatment because, found hope in Dr. Chamria's expertise in zygomatic implants. This taught the importance of continuous learning and

perseverance. This case demonstrated Dr. Chamria's commitment to staying at the forefront of dental technology. His willingness to learn and adopt new techniques ensured that his patients received the best possible care, regardless of how challenging their cases were.

- **Resilience:** After a health setback, Dr Chamria's determination saw him return to treating patients within weeks. His recovery underscored the value of willpower and resilience. Dr. Chamria's remarkable recovery and swift return to his practice highlighted his resilience and dedication. This experience reinforced the importance of perseverance and a positive mindset in overcoming life's challenges.

Takeaway Message for Readers

Dr Arun Chamria's story is a powerful reminder of the importance of passion, perseverance, and compassion. His journey from a small village in Rajasthan to becoming a celebrated Dentist illustrates the impact of dedication and empathy in healthcare. His innovative practices and commitment to continuous learning offers valuable lessons for anyone aspiring to make a difference.

Dr. Arun's life is a testament to the power of perseverance, innovation, and compassion. From his early decisions to prioritizing long-term goals over immediate opportunities, to his ability to gracefully accept defeat and build lasting relationships, Arun consistently demonstrated humility and dedication. His innovative approach to business and dentistry, combined with his deep sense of responsibility towards family and community, highlights a legacy of resilience and selflessness. Dr. Arun's journey inspires us to pursue excellence with a compassionate heart, making a lasting impact on those around us.

For readers, the key takeaway is that true success in any field is not just about professional achievements but about the impact one makes on others' lives. Dr. Chamria's approach to patient-centred care, his innovative practices, and his commitment to continuous learning serve as valuable lessons for anyone aspiring to make a difference.

Probing Patient Concerns: Foundation of Exceptional Care

In the previous chapter, we delved into the transformative journey of Dr. Arun, a man who turned challenges into opportunities and became a profound dentist. Now, we will explore the first pillar of The Royal Ritual, curated by him which summarises his 40 years of Dental expertise. The first pillar highlights the importance of a patient-centered approach in understanding patient concerns. Building on Dr. Arun's legacy, this chapter emphasizes the critical role of addressing patient worries to provide exceptional dental care. Let's delve into the essential practice of Probing Patient Concerns, the foundation of outstanding dental service.

Pillar 1: Probing Patient Concerns

When Dr. Arun entered medical school, he often shared his fascinating yet intense experiences. One story that stands out involved a biology experiment with a frog. Eager to involve his sisters in his learning journey, he brought home a live frog, secured it on a wooden plank with nails. He performed the dissection to demonstrate his medical skills to his sisters.

Although the lesson was informative, the emotional impact lingered. Seeing the life fade from the frog deeply affected them. Dr. Arun, sensing their distress, assured them that he would never harm another living being for the sake of learning. This experience taught him an invaluable lesson: the importance of empathy and understanding the emotional concerns of others.

This lesson carried forward into his dental practice. Dr. Arun understood that patient care goes beyond technical skills. It involves probing patient concerns and addressing their fears and discomforts with compassion. His ability to connect with patients on an emotional level became a cornerstone of his practice, making him not just a skilled dentist but a trusted and caring healthcare provider. This story embodies the first pillar of The Royal Ritual: Probing Patient Concerns, highlighting the profound impact of empathy in exceptional dental care.

This first pillar in dentistry involves understanding and addressing patient concerns. This foundational step is where trust begins, setting the stage for outstanding care. Effective patient-centered care hinges on communication, empathy, and adapting to each patient's unique needs. When one doesn’t know what the other person needs, how will one fulfil the gap.

Where is the Magic?

The true magic of dentistry is not in performing miracles or decorative procedures. It is also not merely in mastering complex surgeries. The real power lies in consistently following a well-curated process. This process has been successfully used for four decades. The perfection does not lie in the results but in the process.

As Dr. Chirag, son of Dr Arun says, "We don't attach ourselves to the result of the treatment. Instead, we attach ourselves to the process, the protocol, and the treatment steps. Ensuring the consistency and repeatability of these steps ensures success in our cases. If I were to focus and keep attention on the result, both success and failure would weigh heavily on my mind. Therefore, it is important to establish protocols and then follow them consistently."

The true magic of dentistry lies not in belonging to an elite club but in consistently following a precise and patient-centered process. High levels of perfection in this process build trust and confidence in patients even before they step into the clinic.

The Importance of First Interaction

For any consultant, the first active interaction with a patient begins with the tele-caller, reception staff, or front desk representative. This initial contact is critical because it is during this moment that the human mind develops confidence or otherwise. This is when the patient decides whether to trust the doctor and clinic.

Creating a unified patient experience from the initial contact is crucial. Every interaction, from a phone call to an in-person visit, should reflect the clinic's values of patient-centered care. This means that every detail, from the way the phone is answered to the ambiance of the waiting room, plays a role in shaping the patient's experience. When done properly, this process transforms ordinary dental visits into extraordinary experiences.

This initial interaction should be brief and precise, focusing on understanding the patient's concerns and motivations. For instance, Patient A seeks help for tooth pain, while Patient B may have crooked teeth with varied reasons for treatment, such as preparing for a wedding or enhancing professional confidence. Identifying the true motivation behind their visit is key.

Dr. Arun Chamria often discussed the concept of DSIM, or Dominant Self Interest Motive. The core idea is that identifying the DSIM is crucial for any meaningful conversation. It represents the primal drive that led the patient to seek consultation. By using language that resonates with the DSIM, a consultant can improve the quality of the conversation, boost likability, and ultimately enhance conversion ratio.

Let's say the patient's DSIM is primarily driven by a desire to look good for their wedding in a few months. Knowing this simple fact during the conversation would help the reception understand needs of patient better, which indirectly make patient have confidence on the clinic.

This method can be applied across various consulting scenarios, whether in healthcare, sales, or customer service. Understanding and appealing to the DSIM ensures that conversations are more meaningful and effective, leading to better outcomes for both the consultant and the client.

By ensuring that every touchpoint with the clinic exudes warmth, professionalism, and a genuine concern for the patient's well-being, trust is built from the very beginning.

This initial phase is foundational for building trust and establishing a strong, positive relationship with the patient.

In summary, the first interaction is where confidence is built or lost. It is the gateway to gaining the patient's trust, making it an indispensable step in the patient-centered approach to dental care. Understanding the DSIM and addressing it effectively ensures that the patient feels understood and valued, setting the stage for a successful and lasting patient relationship.

Moments of Connection

Building strong relationships between staff and patients is the cornerstone of the patient-centered model. In this approach, the true guide for a professional is the clients, in this case, the patients. It is the patients' critiques and experiences that shape the development and improvement of a professional practice. Small gestures can significantly impact patient comfort and satisfaction:

- **Wheelchair Accessibility**: Providing access for patients with mobility issues is not just about legal compliance; it's about ensuring their comfort. Accessibility goes beyond ramps and elevators to encompass all aspects of the patient's visit. From the moment a patient arrives, the ease with which they navigate the clinic sets the tone for their entire experience.

- **Refreshments**: Offering water or tea can make patients feel welcome and reduce their anxiety. These simple gestures create a hospitable environment, turning what could be a stressful visit into a more relaxing experience.

- **Waiting Room Comfort**: A comfortable setting with good lighting and soft music can help ease anxiety. Additional options like magazines or television also make the wait more pleasant.
- **Private Rest Rooms**: Recognizing that patients are often tired and in need of personal space during their rest period led to the creation of private rest rooms. This relaxation contributes significantly to the success of consultations and treatments, as a relaxed patient is more likely to respond positively to care.
- **Language and Communication**: Staff members who can speak the patient's native language can make interactions smoother and less stressful. This is especially critical in diverse communities where language barriers can cause significant anxiety.
- **Multicultural Team**: Having a multicultural team who can cater to patients increases comfort. This consideration shows respect for cultural and personal preferences, making the patient feel more at ease during their visit.
- **Appraisals and Feedback**: Regular feedback meetings to enhance patient care, along with recognizing staff achievements, ensure continuous improvement and team morale. Addressing areas for growth help maintain high standards of care and keep the team motivated.

Patient experiences and critiques have shaped the clinic's improvements. Long treatment durations that extend over months were a significant deterrent for many patients. By reducing the treatment duration to one day, the clinic can now accommodate patients who do not have much time to spare.

Similarly, the fear of dentistry was a major factor, but with a relaxing environment, system-driven procedures, advanced technology, and superior anaesthesia, this fear has been minimized. These adjustments, driven by patient feedback, have greatly enhanced the overall patient experience and the success of consultations.

Active Listening and Empathy

- **Initial Interaction**: The initial call, SMS, or WhatsApp message sets the tone for the patient's experience. Receptionists must listen carefully and note the patient's main concerns, ensuring this first interaction is a positive one. This is crucial in building trust and establishing a strong patient relationship. While many interactions are now automated, such as email or SMS notifications, customizing the approach—like using "Hello" for younger patients and "Namaste" for older ones—can make a significant difference.

- **Understand Dominant Self Interest Motive (DSIM)**: Dr. Arun Chamria emphasized the importance of identifying the Dominant Self Interest Motive (DSIM) during the first interaction. This principle focuses on understanding the primal motivation that led the patient to seek consultation. Identifying these motivations helps tailor the consultation and treatment plan to address the patient's core concerns effectively.

- **Resolving Concerns in Detail**: Thoroughly addressing patient concerns assures them that their issues are genuine and will be properly handled. Taking the time to understand their concerns and offering clear explanations can reduce anxiety and build confidence in the care provided. Patients who feel heard tend to experience fewer complications, make fewer complaints, and are more likely to appreciate their consultant.
- **Prioritizing Patient Queries**: Addressing complaints based on their severity ensures that patients feel acknowledged and that their concerns are taken seriously. This approach helps manage time effectively, ensuring that urgent issues are addressed promptly while also keeping other patients informed and comfortable.

Understanding patient concerns is the foundation of trust and maintaining good care. Active listening involves not just hearing the message but also recognizing the feelings and issues conveyed. Simple phrases like, "I understand this can be stressful, but we're here to help," can make a world of difference.

In summary, active listening and empathy form the bedrock of patient-centered care. By focusing on the initial interaction, understanding the patient's DSIM, thoroughly addressing concerns, and prioritizing patient queries, clinicians can build a strong, trust-based relationship with their patients. This approach not only enhances patient satisfaction but also contributes to the overall success of the consultation and treatment process.

Evolution: Traditional to Modern Dentistry

The shift from traditional to modern dentistry has brought significant improvements. But this did not happen very recently, infact India's first light cure composite back in 1980s. Dr Arun had been investing in tools and equipment's since the very beginning of his dental practice.

Lately, many advanced diagnostic services such as CBCT, 3D Printing, CAD-CAM and Scanning; are available in-house, saving patients time and reducing the need for multiple appointments. This integration exemplifies the patient-centred model.

Experience – Comfort – Trust

Navratri was a magical time for Arun's sisters. The nine days of festivities meant colourful garba dances and endless fun with friends. Arun's father, however, had a strict rule: "You can only stay out until 9:30 pm only if Arun, stayed with you both."

"Bhaiya, can we stay just a little longer to dance?" sisters would plead each night. On the ninth night, Arun had a different plan. "Tonight, I really want to see the burning of Ravan," he told his sisters. Watching the end of evil is something special always. This symbolizes the victory of good over evil. It's a powerful reminder that truth and righteousness always prevail.

When they returned home late, their father was waiting, ready to scold them. Arun stood tall and spoke honestly, "Papa, we stayed to watch the burning of evil and feel the victory of good." Their father's eyes softened. Though upset, he respected Arun's honesty. "Next time, inform me if you're going to be late."

Arun's sisters admired her brother's integrity. Despite potential consequences, he never lied. This experience taught her the value of honesty and trust. Years later, as Arun reflected on these Navratri nights, he realized how these lessons applied to patient care. Just as he provided comfort and trust to his sister, in his practice, understanding a patient's experiences and being truthful builds a strong foundation of trust and comfort.

The Experiential Value

Dental treatment is inherently technical, and patients often find it challenging to judge the skill of their dentist directly. Instead, what leaves a lasting impression on them is how they felt during their visit. Creating a positive experience from the moment they walk in, through personalized attention and a welcoming environment, is crucial in shaping their perception and satisfaction.

First Impressions Matter

The initial contact with the clinic sets the tone for the entire visit. A warm greeting from the receptionist, a friendly smile, and an inviting atmosphere help ease any anxieties patients might have. Small gestures, like offering a beverage or providing clear directions, can make patients feel valued and respected from the outset.

Personalized Attention

Patients appreciate when they are treated as individuals rather than just another appointment. Personal touches, such as remembering a patient's name, asking about their comfort level, and engaging in light conversation, contribute to a sense of care and personal connection. When patients feel that their specific needs and concerns are being addressed, it builds trust and confidence in the dental team.

Comfortable Environment

The physical environment of the clinic plays a significant role in the patient's experience. Comfortable seating, soothing colours, calming music, and pleasant aromas can help create a relaxing atmosphere. Providing entertainment options, such as magazines, television, or even a kids' play area, can make the waiting time more enjoyable. A well-designed clinic that prioritizes patient comfort can significantly reduce stress and anxiety.

Clear Communication

Effective communication is essential in creating a positive patient experience. Explaining procedures in a simple, understandable manner, answering questions patiently, and providing reassurance can alleviate fears and build confidence. Visual aids, such as diagrams or videos, can help patients better understand their treatment plans. Ensuring that patients are well-informed and comfortable with their choices fosters a sense of empowerment and involvement in their own care.

Attention to Detail

Small details often make a big difference in how patients perceive their visit. Ensuring that the clinic is clean and well-organized, that equipment is modern and functioning properly, and that staff are professional and courteous all contribute to a positive experience. Even small gestures, like following up with a phone call after a procedure to check on the patient's well-being, can leave a lasting impression.

Addressing Comfort and Pain Management

One of the biggest concerns for dental patients is pain and discomfort. By employing advanced pain management techniques, offering sedation options, and continuously checking on the patient's comfort during procedures, the dental team can significantly improve the patient's experience. When patients feel that their pain and discomfort are being managed effectively, it enhances their overall perception of care.

Creating Memorable Moments

Memorable moments can turn an ordinary dental visit into an extraordinary one. Celebrating milestones, such as the completion of a long treatment plan, or offering small tokens of appreciation, like a thank-you note or a dental care kit, can make patients feel special. These gestures show that the clinic values their patients and cares about their overall experience.

In summary, the experiential value of a dental visit lies in the holistic approach to patient care. By focusing on creating a welcoming environment, providing personalized attention, maintaining clear communication, paying attention to details, managing comfort effectively, and creating memorable moments, dental clinics can ensure that patients leave with a positive and lasting impression. This not only enhances patient satisfaction but also fosters loyalty and encourages word-of-mouth referrals, contributing to the long-term success of the practice.

The Comfort Factor

Long queues, extended treatment times, and fear of pain are major deterrents in dentistry. Addressing these issues head-on by creating a comfortable and efficient environment can significantly enhance patient satisfaction and trust.

One of the biggest frustrations for patients is waiting for their appointment. Long queues can increase anxiety and discomfort, making the dental visit an unpleasant experience. By adopting an efficient scheduling system and ensuring that appointments run on time, clinics can minimize wait times. One of the core values adopted by Dr Chamria was that he always insisted on an empty waiting room. This can be achieved through:

- **Efficient Appointment Scheduling**: Using advanced scheduling software to manage appointments effectively, ensuring that there are no overlaps and that each patient gets the required attention without unnecessary delays.

- **Staggered Appointments**: Implementing staggered appointment slots to avoid crowding in the waiting area, thereby reducing wait times and enhancing the overall patient experience.

Implementing Same-Day Dentistry

Extended treatment times, requiring multiple visits, can be a significant inconvenience for patients. Implementing same-day dentistry, where possible, can greatly enhance patient convenience and satisfaction. This can be achieved by:

- **Advanced Technology**: Utilizing state-of-the-art technology such as CAD/CAM systems, 3D printers, and digital imaging to perform treatments like crowns, veneers, and restorations in a single visit.

- **Streamlined Processes**: Developing streamlined processes that allow for efficient treatment planning and execution, reducing the need for multiple appointments.

Availability of Senior Doctors

Patients often feel more secure when they know that experienced professionals are readily available. Ensuring the availability of a senior doctor round the clock, at least over a phone call, can provide immense reassurance to patients. This can be facilitated by:

- **On-Call Availability**: Having a senior doctor available for phone consultations to address any urgent concerns or complications, offering patients peace of mind knowing that expert advice is just a call away.

- **Emergency Appointments**: Providing options for emergency appointments, ensuring that patients can receive timely care in critical situations.

Prioritizing Patient Comfort

Patient comfort should be at the forefront of any dental practice. Creating an environment that prioritizes comfort can alleviate fears and build confidence. This involves:

- **Comfortable Environment**: Designing the clinic with patient comfort in mind, including comfortable seating, pleasant decor, calming music, and a welcoming atmosphere.
- **Pain Management**: Employing advanced pain management techniques and offering sedation options to ensure that procedures are as pain-free as possible.
- **Patient-Centric Care**: Continuously checking on the patient's comfort during procedures, offering breaks if needed, and providing clear communication to keep them informed and at ease.

Building Confidence and Credibility

Patients appreciate efficiency and care that respect their time and alleviate their fears. By addressing these key areas, clinics can build confidence and credibility:

- **Respect for Time**: Demonstrating respect for the patient's time by minimizing wait times and offering efficient, high-quality care. This shows that the clinic values the patient's schedule and prioritizes their convenience.
- **Transparent Communication**: Providing clear and transparent communication about treatment plans, procedures, and any potential discomfort. This helps build trust and ensures that patients feel informed and involved in their care.
- **Consistent Quality**: Maintaining a consistent level of high-quality care through standardized procedures and continuous improvement. This reliability builds credibility and encourages patient loyalty.

The Trustworthiness

At Taj Hotels, the staff is trained to never say "no" to a client, embodying the pinnacle of patient service. This technique, if incorporated into dental practice, can elevate patient comfort to the highest level. The philosophy is that it is not the most capable but the most acceptable who wins.

By adopting this approach in a dental clinic, staff members are trained to find solutions rather than deny requests. For example, if a patient needs an urgent appointment, instead of saying, "We are fully booked," the staff can say, "Let me see what I can do to accommodate you." This attitude of always finding a way to say "yes" ensures that patients feel valued and understood, significantly enhancing their comfort and satisfaction.

In summary, by eliminating long queues, implementing same-day dentistry, ensuring the availability of senior doctors, prioritizing patient comfort, and adopting a "never say no" approach inspired by Taj Hotels, dental clinics can create a supportive and efficient environment. This strategy not only enhances patient satisfaction but also builds confidence and credibility, ultimately fostering long-term patient relationships and contributing to the success of the practice.

Minimizing Distractions for Patients

The attitude of a consultant should be to assist in reducing the distractions of the individual from their daily tasks and to enhance their quality of life. When this is done, you become trustworthy. Trustworthiness is fundamental in building strong patient relationships and is key to fostering referrals and recommendations, as patients share their positive experiences with others.

The thought of dental treatments or any medical procedure is often seen as a necessity and a distraction for patients. Any activity that distracts the individual from their daily routine can lead to frustration. Therefore, if systems in a professional setup are designed such that the client or patient can offload this distraction, it becomes a true benefit for the patient, significantly increasing trustworthiness.

Practical Case: Porsche's 9-Year Service Contract

Consider the example of Porsche cars, which offers a 9-year service-free contract with insurance. This means that from minor repairs and regular maintenance to total damage, everything is covered in this 9-year period. For the patient, this transforms the car from a potential source of stress and distraction into a source of enjoyment and fulfilment. This comprehensive coverage is one reason why Porsche cars are bought at a premium compared to other luxury cars in the segment. This is one of the inspirations why Dr Arun in his practice, implemented the service-free warranty for treatments.

Similarly, offering service-free warranties on the entire treatment and providing reminders for check-ups can offload the stress from patients. In many consultations, Dr. Chamria would reassure patients by saying, "Now the stress of your teeth belongs to me." This approach conveys a strong sense of responsibility and commitment, helping patients feel cared for and secure.

Key Strategies to Enhance Trustworthiness:

- **Comprehensive Care Plans:** Provide inclusive packages covering all aspects of dental treatment, from consultation to follow-up. This ensures patients aren't burdened by unexpected costs or appointments.
- **Regular Reminders:** Use automated systems to remind patients of upcoming appointments and

check-ups, keeping them engaged with their dental health and showcasing the clinic's proactive care.

- **Transparent Communication:** Offer clear information on treatment plans, costs, and outcomes. Transparent communication fosters trust and ensures patients are well-informed.
- **Aftercare Services:** Provide thorough aftercare, including follow-up calls and checks, to ensure patient satisfaction and recovery, strengthening long-term relationships.
- **Stress-Free Guarantees:** Offer guarantees for certain treatments, like a warranty on dental implants or cosmetic procedures, to provide patients with peace of mind and assurance of quality.

Building Trust Through Empathy and Reliability

Trustworthiness is further enhanced when consultants genuinely empathize with their patients. By recognizing the inherent stress and distraction associated with dental treatments, and by creating systems that alleviate these concerns, consultants can significantly enhance patient satisfaction. This approach not only improves the patient's experience but also elevates the overall perception of the dental practice.

In summary, the goal is to transform dental care from a source of stress into a seamless, supportive aspect of the patient's life. By implementing comprehensive care plans, providing regular reminders, maintaining transparent communication, offering robust aftercare, and providing stress-free guarantees, dental practices can build unparalleled trust and loyalty among their patients. This trust leads to natural referrals and recommendations, as satisfied patients share their positive experiences with others, further enhancing the practice's reputation and success.

Case Studies: Patient-Centered Care in Action

Case Study 1: The Anxious Teenager

A teenager with severe dental anxiety was scheduled for a complex dental procedure.

Approach:

- **Personalized Interaction**: The dentist took extra time to sit with the teenager and their parent before the procedure, explaining each step in simple terms and addressing all concerns.
- **Comfort Measures**: The teen was allowed to listen to their favourite music during the treatment to help distract and calm them.
- **Supportive Environment**: The clinic provided a stress ball and a comforting blanket, ensuring the teenager felt secure. Also offered conscious sedation treatment options for their treatment.

Outcome: The teenager's anxiety was significantly reduced, and the procedure was completed smoothly. The patient and their parent left the clinic feeling satisfied and grateful for the compassionate care, resulting in positive feedback and a new level of trust in the dental practice.

Case Study 2: The Busy Professional

A working professional needed a dental procedure but had a tight schedule.

Approach:

- **Efficient Scheduling**: The clinic arranged an early morning appointment to accommodate the patient's work commitments.
- **Same-Day Dentistry**: Utilizing advanced technology, the necessary procedures were completed in a single visit including scanning, treatment and fixing of teeth.
- **Convenience**: During short breaks in the procedure, the clinic provided a quiet space for the patient to make work calls.

Outcome: The patient managed their work commitments without compromising their dental health. The efficiency and consideration shown by the clinic enhanced the patient's trust and satisfaction, leading to a positive review and recommendations to colleagues.

Case Study 3: The Multilingual Patient

A patient who spoke little English was apprehensive about communicating their dental issues.

Approach:

- **Language Support**: The clinic identified a staff member who spoke the patient's native language and facilitated the consultation in that language.
- **Clear Communication**: Visual aids and simple explanations were used to ensure the patient fully understood their treatment options. Shared before after of other patients to make the patient at ease and feel relatable.
- **Comfort Measures**: Extra time was spent to ensure the patient felt understood and comfortable throughout the visit.

Outcome: The patient felt respected and well-cared-for, leading to a successful treatment and a strong bond with the clinic. This approach also showcased the clinic's commitment to inclusivity and comprehensive care.

Case Study 4: The Elderly Patient

An elderly patient with difficulty walking required dental care.

Approach:

- **Personal Assistance**: Staff members personally escorted the patient from the entrance to the treatment room and back on a wheelchair.
- **Transportation Arrangements**: The clinic arranged a taxi for the patient's return home to ensure their comfort and safety.

- **Patient Comfort**: Extra care was taken to make the treatment as gentle and painless as possible, considering the patient's mobility issues.

Outcome: The patient felt valued and supported, turning a potentially difficult visit into a positive experience. The patient's family expressed their gratitude, leading to increased trust and further referrals.

Case Study 5: The Pre-Wedding Smile Makeover

A young woman wanted her teeth straightened before her wedding in a few months.

Approach:

- **Tailored Treatment Plan**: The dentist designed a treatment plan that could achieve significant improvement within the given timeframe.
- **Advanced Techniques**: Fast-acting orthodontic options and cosmetic procedures were utilized to enhance her smile efficiently.
- **Continuous Support**: The clinic provided regular updates and support to ensure the patient remained confident and stress-free throughout the process.

Outcome: The patient achieved a beautiful smile in time for her wedding, boosting her confidence. She appreciated the clinic’s dedication and personalized care, resulting in heartfelt testimonials and referrals from her family and friends.

Summary

These case studies illustrate the impact of a patient-centered approach in dentistry. By addressing individual needs, providing personalized care, and creating a supportive environment, dental practices can significantly enhance patient satisfaction, build trust, and foster long-term relationships.

Analysing & Dismantling Problems: Precision in Diagnosis

In the previous chapter, we explored the importance of probing patient concerns as the foundation of exceptional care. Now, we delve into the second pillar of dentistry in The Royal Ritual: Analysing & Dismantling Problems. This pillar is all about precision in diagnosis, a cornerstone of effective treatment. Building on active listening and empathy, this chapter emphasizes the critical role of accurate diagnosis in creating successful treatment plans, highlighting the collaborative effort between dentists and patients.

Pillar 2: Analysing & Dismantling Problems

Dr Arun was a natural teacher, especially adept at simplifying complex subjects like geography and math. Under his guidance, his younger siblings excelled, scoring impressively in subjects. His methodical approach not only helped family members but extended to his deep passion for reading. He once astonished everyone by reading four books, including Dale Carnegie's "How to Win Friends and Influence People," in just four hours.

Known for his photographic memory, he could recall details effortlessly. His real talent, however, lay in his ability to break down problems methodically. He would dissect issues, finding solutions by analysing them from various angles. This skill wasn't just academic; it extended to everyday challenges, teaching valuable lessons in diagnosis and problem-solving.

Reflecting on his approach, it becomes clear that his methods emphasize the importance of thorough analysis, systematic dismantling of problems, and a patient, methodical mindset. These principles are crucial in fields like patient care, where understanding complexities and methodically approaching issues leads to effective diagnosis and treatment strategies.

Precision in Diagnosis

The journey towards an effective treatment, begins with a precise diagnosis. This involves not only listening to the patient but also interpreting their symptoms accurately. Often, patients may struggle to describe their issues, and it is the dentist's role to provide clarity. Simply naming the problem can offer significant emotional and mental relief, setting the stage for successful treatment.

Precision in diagnosis and effective problem analysis are critical aspects of exceptional dental care. Dr Arun mentions how this approach begins with a thorough examination and understanding of each patient's unique needs and concerns. Accurate diagnosis is fundamental to identifying the root causes of dental issues and crafting tailored treatment plans.

For example, when dealing with complex cases like cracked or broken teeth, he always employed advanced diagnostic tools such as X-rays even back in early 2000s to assess the extent of damage accurately. This detailed analysis ensures that the underlying problems are identified and addressed, whether it involves performing a root canal to save a severely damaged tooth or deciding on dental reconstruction options.

Patients' relief and gratitude upon receiving accurate diagnoses

A patient once visited a local dentist in the south of India, carrying his X-rays. Upon examining the X-rays, the local dentist immediately recognized the complexity of the treatment that was performed. He remarked, "There is only one dentist in India who can perform this level of treatment in a single day, and that dentist is in Mumbai."

This statement highlights the critical importance of precision in diagnosing dental issues. The ability to accurately analyse a patient's details is crucial, as it opens many aspects related to the patient's health and overall well-being. This story reveals how meticulous attention Dr Arun gave for his patient work which was known in the dental fraternity.

This anecdote emphasizes the significance of a detailed, patient-focused approach in dental care. It showcases how a thorough analysis and dismantling of dental problems can lead to precise, effective treatments, setting a high standard in the field of dentistry.

Power of Accurate Diagnosis

Accurate diagnosis is the cornerstone of exceptional dental care. It involves a combination of careful listening, thorough examination, and the use of advanced diagnostic tools. This chapter highlights how a detailed consultation, virtual dental consultations, and multiple treatment plans contribute to precise diagnosis and patient satisfaction.

Detail Consultation: The first step in diagnosing a dental issue is a comprehensive consultation. This involves listening to the patient's concerns, examining their medical history, and conducting a detailed physical examination. A thorough consultation allows the dentist to gather all necessary information and provides a foundation for accurate diagnosis.

Virtual Dental Consultation: In today's digital age, virtual consultations have become an invaluable tool. They allow patients to discuss their concerns with a dentist remotely, making dental care more accessible. Virtual consultations also enable patients to seek second opinions and explore treatment options without the need for an in-person visit.

Multiple Treatment Plans and Options: Offering multiple treatment plans ensures that patients have choices and can select the option that best suits their needs and preferences. This collaborative approach fosters trust and ensures that patients feel involved in their care.

Stories of Relief and Gratitude

Patients often experience immense relief and gratitude upon receiving accurate diagnoses and effective treatment plans. Here are a few stories that illustrate the impact of precision in diagnosis:

Persistent Toothache: A patient came in with a persistent toothache that had been misdiagnosed several times. After a detailed consultation and a thorough examination, Dr. Arun Chamria identified that the pulp of the tooth was hyperaemic due to abnormal biting forces. By simply polishing the tooth and slightly reducing its height, the balance was restored, and the pain vanished. The patient was relieved to finally understand the cause of their pain and was grateful for the accurate diagnosis and effective treatment.

Complex Orthodontic Case: A young patient with a complex orthodontic issue had been advised to undergo extensive surgery. Seeking a second opinion, they visited the clinic. Dr. Chamria used advanced diagnostic tools to analyse the problem and developed a less invasive treatment plan. The patient and their family were overjoyed with the alternative solution and the expertise provided.

Home-maker with Swollen Gums: A long-time patient of Dr. Arun suffered persistent tooth pain and swollen gums despite repeated treatments. Suspecting an underlying issue, Dr. Arun reviewed her blood reports and identified elevated thyroid levels. He advised her to seek medical treatment for her thyroid, which ultimately resolved her dental issues. This case exemplifies Dr. Arun's holistic approach and precision in diagnosis, highlighting the importance of considering a patient's overall health for effective treatment.

Elderly Patient’s Indigestion: An elderly patient experienced regular indigestion and was taking antacids daily. This was due to missing teeth, preventing proper chewing of food. By providing the patient with new chewing teeth, the acid reflux and indigestion were greatly reduced. The patient's quality of life improved dramatically, demonstrating the power of an accurate diagnosis.

Precision in Diagnosis: Story of Expertise & Trust

In early 2012, a patient diagnosed with oral cancer sought the expertise of Dr. Arun, a renowned dental surgeon. Although Dr. Arun was not yet qualified to perform oral cancer surgery, his deep understanding of the anatomy of the head and neck allowed him to precisely outline a surgical plan that could potentially save the patient's jaw.

Impressed by Dr. Arun's detailed and accurate plan, the patient took it to his oral surgeon and requested it be considered. After reviewing the plan, the oral surgeon agreed to proceed exactly as Dr. Arun had suggested. The surgery was a success, preserving the patient's jaw and significantly improving his quality of life.

This experience cemented the patient’s trust in Dr. Arun and his team's ability to diagnose with precision. To this day, the patient and his family continue to visit Dr. Arun for their dental care, confident in the meticulous and expert attention they receive.

Dr. Arun's story highlights the critical importance of precision in diagnosis. His ability to analyse complex cases and provide detailed, actionable plans not only showcases his expertise but also builds lasting trust with his patients. This commitment to precision and patient care is a cornerstone of his practice, ensuring that every patient receives the best possible treatment tailored to their unique needs.

Active Listening: Listening to the patient's concerns is the first step in understanding their problems. By actively listening, dentists can gather valuable information that may not be immediately apparent through examination alone.

Medical History and Examination: Reviewing the patient's medical history and conducting a thorough examination are essential for accurate diagnosis. This process helps identify underlying issues that may contribute to the patient's symptoms.

Reading and Staying Current: Keeping abreast of the latest research and developments in dentistry is vital. Dr. Arun Chamria's dedication to continuous learning, inspired by the wisdom of experts like Dr. Donald Bentley, ensures that the clinic remains at the forefront of dental care.

Advanced Technology and Equipment: Integrating advanced technology into the diagnostic process enhances accuracy and efficiency. Tools such as digital X-rays, 3D model printing, and surgical guides provide detailed insights that are crucial for precise diagnosis.

Digital X-rays, 3D Printing: These technologies allow for a more detailed and accurate view of dental structures, aiding in the diagnosis of complex issues.

Surgical Guides: These tools help plan and execute precise surgical procedures, ensuring better outcomes for patients.

Emphasizing Patient Choice and Comfort

The treatment planning process prioritizes patient choice and comfort. By offering multiple treatment options and involving patients in decision-making, the clinic ensures that each patient receives personalized care tailored to their needs.

Patient-Centric Approach: A patient-centric approach involves understanding the patient's preferences and concerns, and incorporating them into the treatment plan. This fosters a sense of trust and collaboration, making the patient feel valued and heard.

Effective Communication: Clear and empathetic communication is essential in discussing diagnosis and treatment options. Ensuring that patients fully understand their diagnosis and the proposed treatment plans helps them make informed decisions and feel more confident in their care.

Precision in diagnosis is fundamental to exceptional dental care. By combining active listening, thorough examination, advanced technology, and continuous learning, the clinic ensures accurate diagnoses and effective treatment plans. The collaborative effort between dentists and patients, coupled with a patient-centric approach, creates a positive and empowering experience for every patient. As we continue to build on the pillars of exceptional care, the commitment to accuracy and empathy remains at the heart of our practice, ensuring that each patient receives the highest standard of care.

Decision Fatigue and its Consequences

Dr. Arun had a unique approach to his daily routine that often led to debates with his wife. She enjoyed showering him with clothes of different colours and styles, but he always preferred white. This habit, which he maintained throughout his life, was to avoid decision fatigue. By eliminating the daily choice of what to wear, he believed he could conserve mental energy for more important tasks, such as his dental practice and patient care.

His friends often teased him about his predictable wardrobe, calling him "the man in white." One day, a close friend asked him, "Arun, why do you always wear white? Don't you get bored?" Dr. Arun smiled and replied, "It's about simplicity and focus. By wearing white every day, I remove one small decision from my life, freeing my mind to concentrate on my work and my patients. Plus, white represents cleanliness and purity, important in our profession."

Research suggests that the average person makes about 35,000 decisions each day. These decisions range from trivial choices like what to eat for breakfast to significant ones like career moves or financial investments. Among these, the most relevant decisions are related to finances, career, and health. Others, like those involving relationships, food, entertainment, travel, and routine, are often considered less critical. For a dentist, prioritizing patient care is paramount, exemplifying the concept of decision fatigue, which affects everyone constantly.

Dr. Arun's simplicity in attire mirrored his professional approach. Just as he removed the decision of what to wear, he methodically dismantled and analysed complex dental issues. He broke down each case into fundamental components, ensuring a thorough understanding before proceeding with a diagnosis or treatment plan.

Importance of Recording Patient Concerns

Listening to patient concerns is crucial, but recording this information is equally important for accurate diagnosis and effective care. Without proper documentation, valuable details can be lost, rendering the information irrelevant.

Establishing a Standard Operating Procedure (SOP) for documentation is essential. Start by noting the current process during patient interactions and consultations. Continuously refine and update these procedures based on feedback and new insights. Although initially time-consuming, this approach leads to significant improvements over time.

An effective SOP ensures no critical information is overlooked, fosters systematic care, and strengthens patient trust. Ongoing refinement of the SOP helps the practice adapt to new challenges, ultimately enhancing patient outcomes and satisfaction.

Application in Dental Practice

In many consultations, Dr. Chamria would reassure patients by saying, "Now the stress of your teeth belongs to me." This approach conveys a strong sense of responsibility and commitment, helping patients feel cared for and secure. Similarly, offering written diagnosis and treatment options, one can offload the stress from patients.

Key Strategies to Enhance Problem Diagnosis:

1. **Comprehensive Check-ups:** Offering inclusive care packages that cover all aspects of dental treatment, from initial consultation to follow-up care including scans. This can include medical history, dental history, X-rays and scan, blood reports, photos etc.

2. **Regular Reminders:** Engage in active listening to understand patient symptoms and concerns fully. Ask open-ended questions to gather more in-depth information about the patient's condition and keep them on record.

3. **Holistic Approach:** Consider the patient's overall health, lifestyle, and psychological factors that may influence their condition. Look beyond the immediate symptoms to understand underlying causes and contributing factors. Consult with other specialists when necessary to gain additional insights.

4. **Utilize Technology:** Implement diagnostic software and artificial intelligence to assist in identifying patterns and anomalies. Leverage telemedicine for remote consultations and second opinions.

5. **Written Approach:** Seek robust training from seniors, including follow-up of patients, to ensure overall learning and ensure the discussions are clear to the patient verbally and in writing.

Summary

In Dr. Arun's approach to dentistry, precision in diagnosis is paramount. He combines active listening with methodical problem-solving skills to ensure accurate identification of dental issues. This method not only alleviates patient concerns but also forms the basis for effective treatment plans tailored to each individual. Dr. Arun's commitment to thorough examination, advanced diagnostic tools, and a patient-centric approach highlights his expertise in dismantling complex dental problems. His holistic approach, supported by continuous learning and empathy, sets a high standard in dental care, ensuring every patient receives personalized and exceptional treatment.

Tracing Roots Cause: Unveil the Underlying Issues

In the previous chapter, we explored the significance of precise diagnosis in dental care. Now, we move to the third pillar of dentistry in The Royal Ritual: Tracing Root Causes. This pillar focuses on understanding the underlying issues that lead to dental problems, ensuring that treatments are not just effective but also preventive. By tracing root causes, dental professionals can provide holistic care that addresses the origins of dental conditions, offering patients long-term solutions and peace of mind.

Pillar 3: Tracing Root Cause: Unveil the Underlying Issues

When Dr Arun was young, he often found comfort sleeping on the sofa in their cosy home. It was when he got married that he witnessed a poignant lesson in compassion and generosity. A carpenter named Mohammed, a frequent visitor for household repairs, was working on the room furniture for Arun and his wife. One day, he broke down in tears, and being concerned, his family inquired about the cause of his distress. Mohammed explained his urgent need for Rs. 5000 to save his struggling shop and support his family, fearing he might have to leave Mumbai without this capital.

Known for his benevolent spirit and disciplined life, Arun's father swiftly retrieved an envelope containing the amount he required, a significant portion of his earnings. He insisted Mohammed take the money, reassuring him to repay whenever possible. Gratefully, Mohammed vowed to repay the kindness by crafting the finest furniture for their home.

That evening, Arun's wife voiced concern over the substantial sum given away, mindful of their own financial constraints. However, he responded with a joyful heart, affirming, "It's our duty to help those in need. He needed it more than we did." This act of selfless giving left an indelible mark on everyone. True to his promise, Mohammed diligently created exquisite furniture for their home over the following year, refusing any payment for his labour. When he finally repaid the loan, he humbly expressed, "I can never repay your kindness. I am here today because of you. Let me do this little."

This story became a cornerstone of Dr. Arun's values, instilling in him the principles of compassion, generosity, and understanding the needs of others. It shaped his approach to patient care and community service, emphasising the importance of tracing the root cause of someone's struggles and offering meaningful assistance where it's most needed.

Exploring a patient's dental issues often unfolds like a detective story. Clues are gathered, and revelations are made that lead to a deeper understanding of their oral health problems. These investigations guide dental professionals not just to treat but to resolve the underlying causes of dental conditions.

Sharing Narratives of Patients' Journeys

Understanding the root causes of dental problems is essential for providing comprehensive care. Here are three distinct case studies that highlight the importance of tracing root causes in dental care:

Case Study: Mystery of Recurring Decay

A 35-year-old elementary school teacher faced a perplexing situation. Despite adhering to a stringent oral hygiene routine and making multiple visits to Dr Arun, she battled with recurring dental decay. Her frustration was palpable, as each visit seemed to conclude with the discovery of new cavities.

Initially, her treatments focused solely on addressing the cavities as they were identified—filling each one in the hope it would be the last. However, the recurring nature of her problem prompted Dr Arun and the team to look deeper. A comprehensive review of her dental history, lifestyle, and tests led to a surprising discovery: Patient has severe gastric reflux issues and for that she practises yoga in which she is supposed to regurgitate. This in turn increases the acidity in her mouth, thereby accelerating tooth decay.

Armed with this knowledge, Dr Arun Chamria tailored a specific treatment plan that included diet and a prescription fluoride treatment alongside her regular hygiene routine. She was also advised on dietary changes to help manage the acidity in her mouth. This holistic approach not only curtailed the formation of new cavities but also equipped her with the knowledge to prevent future issues, transforming her role from a passive recipient of care to an active participant in her dental health.

Case Study: Unexplained Gum Bleeding

A 40-year-old software developer experienced persistent gum bleeding, which he initially dismissed as the result of brushing too hard. However, when the bleeding did not subside, he sought professional help. Initial examinations suggested mild gingivitis, and he was treated accordingly. But the bleeding continued, baffling the entire team of Dr Arun.

Further investigation was warranted. He underwent a series of comprehensive evaluations that included blood tests, a dietary review, and a detailed discussion of his medical history. It was during this thorough scrutiny that diabetes was diagnosed, which is often associated with an increased risk of periodontal diseases. His gum bleeding was a symptom of his undiagnosed diabetes as much as it was of any dental condition.

His treatment plan was adjusted to address both his periodontal condition and his diabetes. He was referred to an endocrinologist to manage his diabetes, while his dental care was tailored by Dr Arun, which included more frequent cleanings and specific periodontal treatments. The dual approach not only alleviated his symptoms but also significantly improved his overall health.

Moments of Clarity and Empowerment

Ten years into marriage, he was blessed with two little angels and a charming boy. Family duties kept his wife busy as a homemaker while he focused on his clinic. However, as the demands of his professional life grew, it became clear that both management and clinical decisions required more attention.

To avoid decision fatigue, as previously discussed, and to have a trusted family member involved, he convinced his wife to join him at the clinic. This way, the children would learn to be more self-reliant, and the clinic would flourish under his wife's guidance. By tracing the root cause of their need for growth and trust, they successfully integrated family and professional life, ensuring both thrived.

Empowerment stems from both taking responsibility and having the authority to act. Throughout Dr. Arun's life, he has experienced and provided this empowerment, a practice that holds valuable lessons for clinical practice and business alike. Identifying gaps and addressing them effectively is crucial for success in any field.

In clinical practice, patient empowerment is fundamental. Dr. Arun believes that patients should be involved in their treatment decisions, including choosing their doctor and deciding on payment methods. This active participation fosters a sense of ownership and confidence in their care, leading to better health outcomes and higher satisfaction.

For healthcare providers, clarity and empowerment come from understanding their roles and responsibilities. Dr.

Arun's approach ensures that his team knows precisely what steps to take and how to execute them. This clarity reduces ambiguity, enhances efficiency, and ensures that the highest standards of care are maintained.

In the business realm, empowerment involves informed decision-making. For investors, this means understanding which shares to invest in based on thorough research and analysis. Dr. Arun applies this principle to his practice, ensuring that every investment in technology, infrastructure, and training is strategically planned and executed.

Dr. Arun's life is a testament to the power of clarity and empowerment. By identifying and bridging gaps, whether in patient care or business strategy, he has created an environment where everyone involved—patients, healthcare providers, and stakeholders—feels confident and capable. This holistic approach not only drives success but also fosters a culture of continuous improvement and innovation.

The journey toward dental health is significantly enhanced when patients are actively involved in their treatment decisions. This empowerment comes from moments of clarity that occur when patients fully understand their dental conditions and the treatment options available to them. Such moments are transformative, turning passive recipients of healthcare into active participants who are engaged and motivated to maintain their dental health.

Tracing the Root Cause: With Knowledge

In the realm of dentistry, Dr. Arun Chamria embodies the principle of tracing the root cause with a profound emphasis on knowledge. This approach stems from his early experiences, notably a lesson learned from his teachers. The education and interaction-based approach laid the foundation for Dr. Arun's understanding towards patient care and the need to delve deeper into their concerns.

Dr. Arun's commitment to knowledge involves thorough patient consultations and comprehensive examinations. He believes that a holistic understanding of a patient's dental history, medical conditions, and lifestyle factors is essential for accurate diagnosis and effective treatment planning. This approach not only ensures that symptoms are properly managed but also aims to prevent recurring issues by addressing their root causes. By continuously expanding his knowledge through research, seminars, and collaboration with peers, Dr. Arun ensures that he remains adept at identifying and treating complex dental conditions at their source.

Through his practice, Dr Arun exemplifies how tracing the root cause with knowledge can lead to better patient outcomes and enhance overall dental health. His dedication to understanding the complete picture of each patient's oral health journey underscores his belief that informed decisions based on thorough analysis are key to providing exceptional dental care.

Tracing through Technology

In the modern landscape of dental care, Dr Arun integrates advanced technology seamlessly into his practice to trace the root cause of dental issues with precision. Embracing technological advancements such as digital X-rays, 3D imaging, and intraoral cameras, Dr. Arun enhances his diagnostic capabilities to a level previously unattainable. These tools allow him to visualise dental structures and anomalies in intricate detail, facilitating accurate identification of underlying problems.

Digital X-rays, for instance, provide immediate and high-resolution images of teeth and surrounding tissues, aiding in the detection of cavities, fractures, and infections that may not be visible to the naked eye. Likewise, 3D imaging technology offers comprehensive views of dental anatomy, enabling Dr. Arun to plan and execute treatments with unparalleled accuracy. By utilising intraoral cameras during examinations, he ensures that every aspect of a patient's oral health is meticulously documented and assessed.

Beyond diagnosis, Dr. Arun employs technological solutions in treatment planning and patient education. Virtual simulations and CAD/CAM technology enable him to design and fabricate precise dental restorations, from crowns to implants, tailored to each patient's unique anatomy. This personalised approach not only enhances treatment outcomes but also improves patient satisfaction by involving them in the decision-making process.

By leveraging technology, Dr. Arun Chamria exemplifies how tracing the root cause with advanced tools can revolutionise dental care. His integration of cutting-edge technology ensures that patients receive optimal care that is both effective and tailored to their individual needs, setting a new standard for excellence in modern dentistry.

Role of Trust and Communication

Trust and communication are the bedrock of any therapeutic relationship, particularly in dentistry, where anxiety and fear are prevalent. Building strong patient-dentist relationships is essential for effective care.

Modern dental practices equipped with advanced technologies like digital imaging and 3D modelling have revolutionised how dentists communicate issues and treatment plans to their patients. For instance, Dr. Lee utilizes intraoral cameras to show her patients the exact nature of their dental issues in real-time, making abstract conditions tangible. This technology not only aids in precision but also enhances patient trust, as they can visually confirm the diagnosis themselves.

The psychological comfort patients feel when they believe their concerns are understood cannot be overstated. Dr Arun makes it a practice to spend the first part of his consultations simply listening, allowing his patients to express all their concerns and fears without interruption. This practice has led to higher satisfaction rates in his clinic, as patients feel genuinely cared for and valued.

The path to Spirituality

As a young man, Dr Arun Chamria attended a significant pooja at Triyambhakeshwar with his wife, where he received advice not to consume anything given for free after the ceremony. Taking this to heart, he followed this practice diligently for 45 days and later incorporated it into his daily life.

This experience taught him a profound lesson about the root cause of personal and professional challenges: the imbalance between seeking and giving. By refraining from seeking, Dr Arun discovered that he naturally started giving more, realising that this shift in mindset was crucial for personal growth and societal contribution. This practice became symbolic of his belief in addressing the root causes of problems by fostering a balanced approach between receiving and giving in all aspects of life.

Driven by his newfound understanding, Dr Arun Chamria initiated a meaningful practice in the early 2000s of distributing biscuit packets at traffic signals. This initiative aimed not only to prevent children from adopting harmful habits but also to provide them with food, addressing immediate needs within the community.

This simple yet impactful gesture reflects Dr Arun's commitment to tracing the root cause of societal issues—such as hunger and youth vulnerability—and addressing them at their core through thoughtful action. By identifying and acting upon the underlying needs of the community, Dr Arun exemplifies how tracing root causes can lead to meaningful solutions that benefit individuals and society as a whole.

Celebrating the Diverse Skills of Dental Professionals

A successful dental team goes beyond technical proficiency in clinical procedures; it integrates patient comfort with a thorough understanding of root causes for effective treatment. This holistic approach begins with the initial patient consultation, where every aspect of the patient's dental health is meticulously examined and documented. Once the initial diagnosis is made, all relevant reports and findings are recorded for review during the final consultation with Dr Arun Chamria.

During the final consultation, Dr Arun leads a comprehensive examination and discussion with the dental team. This collaborative session allows each member to contribute their expertise and insights based on the patient's condition. By pooling together knowledge and experiences, the team explores various treatment possibilities and develops a tailored plan of action. This collective brainstorming not only enhances diagnostic accuracy but also ensures that all potential avenues for treatment are considered.

The team's discussion generates valuable insights into the underlying causes of the patient's dental issues. This deeper understanding enables them to address not just the symptoms but also the root causes of oral health problems. For example, identifying lifestyle factors, underlying medical conditions, or genetic predispositions that contribute to dental issues allows for a more targeted and effective treatment approach.

Moreover, sharing knowledge and experiences among peers within the team fosters a culture of continuous learning and improvement. Each team member brings a unique perspective to the table, enriching the overall diagnostic and treatment planning process. This collaborative effort not only benefits the patient by ensuring comprehensive care but also enhances the professional growth and development of each team member.

In essence, tracing the root cause in dental care involves a systematic approach of thorough examination, collaborative discussion, and integrated treatment planning. By understanding and addressing the underlying factors contributing to dental problems, the dental team under Dr Arun Chamria's guidance ensures optimal patient outcomes and long-term oral health. This commitment to holistic care exemplifies how tracing root causes leads to more effective and personalised treatments, ultimately improving patient care and satisfaction.

Summary

In "The Royal Ritual," Dr Arun Chamria explores the pivotal role of tracing root causes in dentistry, emphasising a shift from symptomatic treatment to understanding the underlying issues driving dental problems. This approach, inspired by his father's compassionate act towards a struggling carpenter, underscores the importance of addressing the core origins of issues for sustainable solutions. By delving deep into patients' dental histories, lifestyles, and comprehensive examinations, Dr. Arun ensures precise diagnosis and personalised treatment plans that not only alleviate current issues but also prevent future complications. Through this holistic approach, he exemplifies how tracing root causes empowers patients with long-term dental health and enhances overall well-being.

Intuitive Treatment Planning: Crafting Personalized Solutions

In the previous chapter, we explored the significance of tracing root causes to provide effective and preventive dental care. Now, we move to the fourth pillar of The Royal Ritual: Intuitive Treatment Planning. This pillar focuses on crafting personalised solutions that address each patient's unique needs and preferences. Through intuitive treatment planning, dental professionals can offer hope and relief, transforming the patient experience and fostering long-term oral health.

Pillar 4: Intuitive Treatment Planning: Crafting Personalized Solutions

Dr. Arun always emphasized the importance of providing patients with options. When asked why, he explained, "The mind is constantly making decisions. It's crucial to educate patients, and from a medico-legal perspective, no fact should be omitted." This philosophy underscores his commitment to transparency and informed consent.

Dr. Arun's dedication to continuous learning played a significant role in shaping his practice. He regularly referenced books and attended conferences to stay abreast of the latest developments in dentistry. These insights were then used to create comprehensive treatment formats at his clinic, ensuring that every aspect of patient care was thoroughly considered.

An example of Dr. Arun's intuitive thinking involves a mother who visited him after consulting with numerous other dentists. She had pervasive gum issues and financial constraints that prevented her from seeking extensive periodontal treatments. Recognizing that her symptoms might have an underlying cause, Dr. Arun advised her to undergo a blood test. The results revealed that she had anaemia. By simply correcting her haemoglobin levels, her gum issues resolved completely.

This case exemplifies Dr. Arun's holistic approach to dental care. His ability to think beyond the obvious and consider the patient's overall health demonstrates the essence of intuitive thinking in dental practice. By looking for root causes and educating patients, Dr. Arun not only resolves immediate dental issues but also promotes long-term well-being.

Dr. Arun's approach to patient care is a testament to the importance of comprehensive, informed, and intuitive decision-making in dentistry. By empowering patients with knowledge and considering their overall health, he ensures that each treatment plan is both effective and personalized, setting a high standard for dental professionals everywhere.

What is intuition in Dentistry?

Intuitive treatment planning in dentistry involves repeating steps so many times that there is a finesse in the work executed. It’s not just about knowledge but also about intuition, which helps with clarity. Repeating diagnostic and treatment procedures countless times helps build an intuitive grasp of clinical situations, leading to more efficient and effective treatment planning.

This approach goes beyond the basics of technical knowledge and clinical skills. It integrates a deep understanding and innate sense of patient needs and conditions, developed through years of experience. This intuition enables quick, accurate decisions even in complex cases, providing a subtle understanding of what might work best for a particular patient.

Intuitive treatment planning also involves a holistic understanding of the patient, including their medical history, lifestyle, and psychological factors. This comprehensive view helps in creating personalized treatment strategies that address the root causes of dental problems, not just the symptoms.

Moreover, an intuitive approach enhances patient communication. Dentist can more effectively explain treatment options, fostering trust and ensuring patients feel more involved in their care decisions. This continuous learning and adaptation process ensures that each patient interaction and treatment experience refines the dentist's intuitive skills and knowledge base.

Intuitive treatment planning is the art of creating individualized care plans that consider the patient's specific conditions, preferences, and lifestyle. This approach ensures that dental treatments are not only effective but also aligned with the patient's expectations and comfort.

Sharing Heart-warming Anecdotes

A New Smile

A 28-year-old marketing executive had always been self-conscious about her misaligned teeth. She avoided smiling in photos and felt insecure in social situations. After consulting with Dr. Arun, she was presented with several treatment options, including braces and ceramic aligners. Concerned about the visibility of traditional braces given her professional role, and with an urgent need to prepare for marriage alliances, she sought a solution that would discreetly straighten her teeth without affecting her appearance.

Understanding her concerns, Dr. Arun recommended a smile beautification treatment that could straighten her teeth in one day. This approach minimized the impact on her professional image while addressing her dental needs efficiently. Throughout the treatment process, she felt supported and confident, knowing that her preferences were respected. The treatment not only improved her smile but also boosted her self-esteem, making her more confident in both her personal and professional life.

Relief for Foreign Patient

A 55-year-old foreign patient, struggled with severe tooth sensitivity and frequent pain. His previous dental treatments provided only temporary relief. Frustrated, he sought a second opinion at Dr Arun's clinic. During his consultation, he shared his concerns and history of treatments. The team conducted a thorough examination and discovered that the underlying issue was worn enamel due to bruxism (teeth grinding).

The personalized treatment plan included custom-made night guards to protect his teeth, along with desensitizing treatments to address the sensitivity. Dr Arun also recommended lifestyle changes to manage stress and to wear a night guard to avoid bruxism. He was overjoyed to finally find a solution where his teeth looked good, and also started to wear nightguard to reduce load on underlying teeth and bone.

Profound Impact of Personalized Care

A patient visited Dr. Arun after consulting several other dentists with no relief, as the X-rays were showing nothing. His younger daughter recollects, as soon as Dr. Arun heard the patient's complaints and did his examination, he was certain of a procedure, despite objections. It was purely his experience and intuition that guided him, resulting in an instant relief for the patient. The patient's words: "Dr. Chamria is not called an authority figure in the field of dentistry for no reason."

Dr. Arun Chamria's approach to dental care emphasizes customized treatment strategies that cater to each patient's unique needs. By understanding that no two patients are alike, he ensures that treatment plans are meticulously tailored to address specific dental concerns while considering individual circumstances such as financial constraints and time availability.

This personalized approach extends beyond merely selecting the right dental procedure; it involves a comprehensive assessment of the patient's oral health history, lifestyle factors, and personal preferences. By offering a range of treatment options and discussing the pros and cons of each, Dr. Arun empowers patients to make informed decisions about their dental care. This thorough customization not only enhances treatment outcomes but also fosters trust and satisfaction among patients, who appreciate the attention given to their individual needs.

The profound impact of personalized care in Dr. Arun Chamria's practice is evident in every aspect of patient interaction and treatment planning. By incorporating patient input at every stage of the process, from initial consultation to final treatment, Dr. Arun ensures that each individual feels valued and understood.

This active involvement in decision-making empowers patients to voice their concerns, preferences, and goals, thereby co-creating a treatment plan that aligns with their expectations. Moreover, by fostering a collaborative relationship built on trust and mutual respect, Dr. Arun enhances the overall patient experience and satisfaction. Patients not only receive expert dental care but also gain a sense of ownership over their oral health journey, leading to long-term benefits in dental health and well-being.

A Collaborative Process of Treatment Planning

Intuitive treatment planning is a collaborative process that involves active participation from both the dentist and the patient. This partnership ensures that treatment plans are tailored to meet the patient's specific needs and preferences.

When you visit your Chartered Accountant, you share your views on income, expenses, and tax distribution. Your CA advises you on ways to reduce taxes. You trust your CA for this expertise. Similarly, you consult a legal lawyer for legal issues. This same principle applies to dental consultants.

Patients come to dentists because they may have trouble with one or a few of their teeth, often not realizing that these issues might be related to other parts of their mouth or even their overall health. As dental professionals, we must serve as the link between dental and overall health, managing patient expectations, especially when they are unrealistic.

More often than not, we have observed that providing patients with a complete picture of their dental and overall health issues brings more clarity. When patients see the full scope of their health concerns, their understanding deepens, and the experiential value of the consultation increases. This comprehensive approach ensures that patients are better informed and more engaged in their treatment plans, leading to improved outcomes and greater satisfaction.

Respecting Patients' Preferences

Personalized treatment planning starts with respecting patient preferences through open communication and shared decision-making. Encourage patients to express their concerns and expectations, which helps tailor a treatment plan that aligns with their goals. For example, some patients may prioritize aesthetics, while others focus on minimizing discomfort or recovery time.

Clear Communication and Transparency

Effective treatment planning requires clear communication and transparency. Dentists should explain the benefits, risks, and expected outcomes of each option in an understandable way. Using visual aids like digital simulations and photos can help patients visualize results. This transparency builds trust and helps patients make informed decisions, including understanding their role in treatment success.

Patient Involvement in Treatment Planning

Active patient involvement in treatment planning ensures they are not passive recipients but active participants. Presenting various options and collaborating on the best fit for their needs and lifestyle can alleviate anxiety and build trust. When patients feel heard and involved, they are more likely to be comfortable and committed to their treatment.

Continuous Feedback and Adjustments

The process doesn’t end with the treatment plan. Continuous feedback and adjustments are crucial to keeping the plan aligned with patient needs. Regular check-ins allow dentists to monitor progress, address concerns, and modify the plan as needed. This flexibility ensures the best care throughout the treatment journey.

Building Long-Term Relationships

Collaborative treatment planning also helps to build long-term relationships between patients and their dental care providers. When patients feel that their needs and preferences are respected, they are more likely to trust their dentist and continue seeking care from them in the future. This trust and continuity of care can lead to better long-term oral health outcomes and a more positive overall experience for the patient.

Transformative Impact of Same-Day Dentistry

Same-Day Dentistry has revolutionized the field, offering patients immediate results and restoring their smiles and confidence in a single visit. This innovative approach exemplifies the principles of intuitive treatment planning by prioritizing convenience, efficiency, and patient satisfaction.

Clear communication and transparency are foundational principles in Dr. Arun Chamria's practice, ensuring that every patient understands their treatment options fully. Each point discussed during consultations is meticulously noted and stored for future reference, reflecting Dr. Arun's commitment to comprehensive care. He believes in openness, providing patients with detailed information about their dental health, proposed treatments, financial considerations, and time commitments. This transparency fosters trust and empowers patients to make informed decisions, supported by documented information shared with them for clarity and informed consent. By prioritizing clear communication, Dr. Arun ensures that patients are actively involved in their dental care journey from start to finish.

Transformative Impact of Same-Day Dentistry

Same-Day Dentistry represents a breakthrough in dental care, allowing Dr. Arun Chamria to restore smiles and confidence swiftly and effectively. Through advanced technology, Dr. Arun can now show patients an approximate preview of their future smile before the treatment begins, a feat previously unimaginable. This capability not only enhances patient satisfaction but also reinstates both smile aesthetics and self-assurance in a single seamless procedure.

Same-Day Dentistry is celebrated for its efficiency and convenience, minimizing the number of visits required while delivering exceptional results. Dr. Arun's expertise in this area exemplifies how technological advancements can revolutionize dental care, offering patients immediate benefits and long-term satisfaction.

Full Mouth Rehabilitation

Dr. Arun's younger daughter recalls her last significant case with her father before starting her own practice. A patient from Pune arrived at 1:45 pm, stating that he would only proceed with the treatment if it could be completed by the next morning. The team sat together, deliberating on how to achieve this daunting task. Dr. Arun confidently said, "If she and I work together, we can do it in 2.5 to 3 hours." True to his word, they completed 30 root canal treatments in just 2.5 hours.

This experience left a lasting impression on everyone involved. The intuition and consistency demonstrated in that moment have become a guiding principle, resonating with Dr. Arun's daughter whenever she faces difficult challenges in her practice.

Summary

Intuitive treatment planning is the cornerstone of personalized dental care. By crafting individualized solutions that respect patients' preferences and needs, dental professionals can provide transformative results that restore smiles and confidence. Clear communication, collaboration, and the innovative approach of Same-Day Dentistry all contribute to the success of personalized treatment plans. As we continue to build on the pillars of exceptional care, the commitment to crafting personalized solutions remains at the heart of our practice, ensuring that every patient receives the highest standard of care tailored to their unique journey.

Executing Treatment with Excellence: Prioritizing Quality Care

In the previous chapters, we have explored the foundational pillars of dentistry, from probing patient concerns to crafting personalised solutions. Now, we turn to the fifth pillar of The Royal Ritual: Executing Treatment with Excellence. This chapter focuses on the commitment to delivering high-quality care during dental procedures, ensuring that every patient experiences the best possible outcomes and leaves the clinic with a smile.

Pillar 5: Executing Treatment with Excellence: Prioritizing Quality Care

When Dr. Arun's younger daughter started her practice in 2011, he insisted she take on multiple roles beyond clinical practice. He had her work in accounts, at the reception, and in human resources, which led to many arguments. As a dentist, she was initially reluctant to embrace these non-clinical roles. Despite her resistance, Dr. Arun paid her a salary based on her work hours in these diverse roles.

She spent ten years as his shadow, and now, after several years into her private practice, she realises the invaluable skills she gained from those experiences. The development of these skills enabled her to set up her online dental shopping platform and grow her private practice independently.

Dr Arun taught her that there is no limit to earning, but it is crucial never to consider one's career small and never to do anything unethical to reach one's goals. This approach instilled a sense of excellence at every step, emphasising the importance of thorough training, ethical practice, and unwavering commitment to patient care. By embracing every role and seeing the best in every situation, she learned to execute treatment with excellence and dedication. Executing patient treatment with excellence means more than just technical proficiency; it encompasses the entire patient experience, from the moment they walk into the clinic to the completion of their treatment.

Opening doors for Foreign Patient Dental Tourism

Dr Arun recalls the challenges faced by international patients back in 2005 when the internet was just gaining traction, and WhatsApp had not yet overtaken SMS as a primary mode of communication. Patients travelling from abroad often struggle with connectivity and communication issues. Recognising these challenges, Dr. Arun collaborated with a travel agency to streamline the process for foreign patients.

This partnership resulted in a comprehensive solution that covered everything from visa approval letters to tickets, travel arrangements, and accommodation. This holistic approach made it possible for patients from over 30 countries to access his clinic with ease. Every detail was meticulously planned, including food preferences, car transport, and even recommendations for places to visit during their stay.

This initiative exemplified the concept of dental tourism, where the entire journey—from obtaining a visa to arriving at the clinic—was seamlessly managed, ensuring a stress-free experience for the patients. Dr. Arun's foresight and dedication to patient care set a new standard in the field, demonstrating that exceptional dental care goes beyond the clinic and encompasses the entire patient experience.

Now imagine if so much was thought for someone travelling all the way thousands of miles, what hospitality would have been offered for those around?

Moments of Joy and Gratitude

The true reward for dental professionals often comes in the form of the joy and gratitude expressed by their patients. These moments of transformation are a testament to the power of exceptional dental care.

From the moment a patient steps into a dental clinic, they should be greeted by warm smiles from well-trained staff members. They might be guided to a private waiting room or taken to the reception to complete paper formalities. Offering a wet towel or refreshments can enhance their experience in terms of comfort and convenience. Simple considerations like whether they are alone or accompanied, or whether they have a chauffeur or are driving themselves, can significantly ease their day.

Even with limited space and resources, dental professionals should strive to fill the emotional gap for patients and create an atmosphere of wellness and care to the point where patients forget they are there for treatment at a dental clinic. Patient comfort, safety, and satisfaction must be the top priorities.

Emphasising Commitment to Excellence

Excellence in dental care is achieved through a combination of skill, knowledge, and a relentless commitment to patient well-being. This commitment is evident in every aspect of treatment, from the techniques used to the overall patient experience.

Advanced Techniques and Technologies

Modern dentistry offers a plethora of advanced techniques and technologies designed to enhance treatment outcomes and patient comfort. For example, the use of laser dentistry allows for minimally invasive procedures with faster healing times and reduced discomfort. Digital imaging provides precise diagnostics, enabling dentists to plan and execute treatments with exceptional accuracy.

The use of digital scanners and CAD/CAM technology to create custom restorations has made dentistry more precise. This technology allows for the design and fabrication of crowns, bridges, and veneers with unparalleled precision, often completed in a single visit. Patients appreciate the convenience and the high-quality results, which reflect a commitment to using the best available tools to enhance patient care. But even without it, the success in treatments was similar to that with it.

Holistic and Comprehensive Care

Excellence in dental treatment also involves taking a holistic approach to patient care. This means considering the patient’s overall health and well-being, not just their dental issues. For instance, a holistic dentist integrates nutrition counselling and stress management techniques into her treatment plans. Dentist believes that oral health is deeply connected to overall health and that addressing lifestyle factors can significantly improve dental outcomes. Patients benefit from this comprehensive approach to Dentistry. The patient's treatment plan has dental and lifestyle changes and not just treatment.

Patient Stories of Joy

One memorable occasion involved an elderly gentleman who had been self-conscious about his smile for decades. His daughter brought him to Dr. Arun's clinic, hoping for a solution. After a series of treatments, the moment arrived when the gentleman looked in the mirror and saw his new smile. Tears welled up in his eyes as he exclaimed, "I never thought I'd see myself smiling like this again." The pure joy on his face was unforgettable, and his daughter, overcome with emotion, hugged her father tightly, expressing her gratitude to Dr. Arun and his team.

Another poignant story features a young woman who had been avoiding social situations due to her misaligned teeth. With an important alliance meeting the next day, she visited

Dr. Arun's clinic in a state of desperation. Understanding the urgency, Dr. Arun and his team worked tirelessly, employing advanced techniques to correct her teeth in a single day. The next morning, she attended her meeting with a radiant smile. Later, she called the clinic, her voice filled with happiness, saying, "He admired my smile! I can't thank you enough." This experience not only boosted her confidence but also opened new doors in her personal life.

These stories highlight the emotional and psychological impact of exceptional dental care. Dr Arun's commitment to providing holistic, patient-centred treatment has led to numerous moments where patients experience tears of joy, renewed confidence, and heartfelt gratitude. Such moments are a powerful reminder of the importance of dental care that goes beyond aesthetics, touching the very essence of a person's self-worth and happiness.

Steps for Effective Dental Consultation Practice

Step 1 Initial Paperwork: Upon a patient's first visit, provide them with a case paper. Ask them to fill in essential details such as Name, Age, Gender, Address, and Occupation. Once completed, the patient should return the form to the receptionist.

Step 2 Case History Recording: The attending dentist should conduct a thorough review, asking several questions to record the patient's history. Even if the patient has previously reported allergies, they should be asked to confirm any existing allergies again to ensure accuracy.

Step 3 Preliminary Examination: Conduct a comprehensive examination and record all necessary details for treatment planning. This includes a thorough inspection of the oral cavity and documenting relevant findings.

Step 4 Diagnostic Imaging: In most cases, an OPG, CBCT, or RVG X-ray investigation is performed to gather detailed imaging before the final consultation.

Step 5 Treatment Options: Explain possible treatment options and plan to the patient, including the advantages and disadvantages of each option. Encourage the patient to ask any relevant questions. Write down the treatment plans on the case paper and provide a copy to the patient.

Step 6 Confirmation and Consent: Ask the patient to confirm their acceptance of the proposed treatment by signing the case paper. Ensure the patient retains a copy for their records. Collect consultancy charges at this stage. Additionally, offer online consultations if needed.

Step 7 Impressions: Take impressions of the patient's single or both jaws as required. Proceed with the plans discussed and agreed upon by the patient.

Step 8 Model Preparation: Begin model preparation within 2-5 minutes of taking the impressions. In about 30 minutes, the patient's teeth model should be ready. Scan the model and feed the computer image into the CAD (Computer-Aided Design) machine for digital teeth design.

Step 9 Digital Design and Machining: Within 30-60 minutes, finalise the design and send it for machining. The CAM (Computer-Aided Manufacturing) machine will prepare the final teeth, taking approximately 10-15 minutes per tooth. Multiple CAM machines are used to prepare the upper and lower jaw teeth simultaneously, reducing the total time by 50%.

Step 10 Patient Comfort: While waiting, ensure the patient and their relatives are comfortable in a waiting room. Offer refreshments to enhance their experience.

Step 11 Anaesthesia and Precautionary Steps: Before the procedure, locally anaesthetise the area to be operated on to ensure numbness during surgery. For dental implants or Zygomatic Implants, take necessary precautionary steps depending on the bone condition to prevent post-operative sensitivity or pain.

Step 12 Final Restoration: In most cases, fix the final restoration on the same day or the next day. In some cases, schedule the fixation for another day if required.

Commitment to Excellence in all aspects of Treatment

Commitment to Excellence: Excellence in dental treatment is not just about achieving the desired clinical outcomes; it's about setting high standards in every aspect of patient care. This includes the initial consultation, the diagnostic process, treatment planning, the execution of procedures, and follow-up care. Every step should reflect a commitment to quality, precision, and patient satisfaction.

Step-Wise Protocol of The Royal Ritual: At The Royal Ritual, each treatment follows a meticulous step-wise protocol designed to ensure the highest standards of care. This protocol begins with a comprehensive assessment of the patient's dental and overall health, followed by a detailed treatment plan tailored to their specific needs. Advanced technologies such as digital imaging and CAD/CAM systems are utilised to enhance accuracy and efficiency, ensuring that treatments are not only effective but also minimally invasive and comfortable for the patient.

Continuous Improvement: The pursuit of excellence involves a commitment to continuous improvement. Dental professionals should regularly update their skills and knowledge through ongoing education and training. This includes attending workshops, seminars, and webinars, as well as staying informed about the latest advancements in dental technology and techniques.

Exceeding Patient Expectations: Exceeding patient expectations requires going above and beyond in every aspect of care. This means not only providing high-quality treatments but also creating a positive and welcoming environment. Patients should feel valued and respected from the moment they enter the clinic. Personalised touches, such as remembering a patient's name and preferences, can significantly enhance their experience and foster long-term loyalty.

Making a Positive Difference in Patients' Lives

One poignant example of this dedication is the story of a foreign patient who visited our clinic for a complex dental procedure. Despite the challenges of travelling and undergoing treatment in a different country, the patient was deeply impressed by the level of care and attention provided. The dental team meticulously planned every aspect of the treatment, ensuring that the patient felt comfortable and well-informed at every step. The patient was so moved by the exceptional care that, upon completion of the treatment, he tipped more than the actual cost of the procedure. This generous gesture was a testament to the profound appreciation he felt for the dedication and professionalism of the dental team.

Oral Health Outcomes

The commitment to excellence at The Royal Ritual directly translates to significant improvements in oral health outcomes for our patients. This is achieved through:

1. **Personalised Care Plans:** Each patient receives a customised treatment plan that addresses their unique needs and conditions.

2. **Preventive Care:** Regular check-ups, cleanings, and patient education about proper oral hygiene practices are integral parts of our preventive strategy.

3. **Advanced Techniques:** Utilization of the latest dental technologies and techniques, such as laser dentistry and CAD/CAM systems, ensures precise and minimally invasive treatments.

4. **Holistic Health Considerations:** Recognizing the connection between oral health and overall health, our dentists incorporate holistic approaches into their treatment plans.

Quality of Treatment

The quality of treatment at The Royal Ritual is reflected in the high satisfaction rates and the positive feedback we receive from our patients. This quality is maintained through:

1. **Skill and Expertise:** Continuous professional development ensures they remain updated with the latest advancements in dentistry.

2. **State-of-the-Art Facilities:** The use of digital imaging, laser dentistry, and other advanced tools enhances the accuracy and quality of care.

3. **Patient-Centric Approach:** This includes personalised care plans, thorough explanations of treatment options, and a warm, welcoming environment.

4. **Continuous Improvement:** Regular training sessions, workshops, and feedback mechanisms help us identify areas for improvement and implement best practices consistently.

5. **Teamwork and Collaboration:** Regular team meetings, open communication, and mutual respect ensure that every team member contributes to providing the best possible care for our patients.

With The Royal Ritual, we believe that the dedication of our dental professionals is the cornerstone of our success. Their commitment to making a positive difference in patients' lives, combined with advanced technology and personalised care, ensures that we provide the highest quality of treatment and achieve outstanding oral health outcomes. Celebrating these achievements reinforces our dedication to excellence and motivates us to continue striving for the best in dental care.

Teamwork and Training: Build a Strong Collaboration

1. Collaborative Dynamics: Effective teamwork and collaboration are essential for achieving excellence in dental care. The HR and staff play a crucial role in creating a cohesive and supportive work environment. Regular team meetings, open communication, and mutual respect are fundamental to fostering a collaborative dynamic.

2. Celebrating Success: Every milestone, no matter how small, is celebrated at The Royal Ritual. Recognising and celebrating achievements boosts team morale and motivation. Whether it's completing a challenging procedure, receiving positive patient feedback, or achieving professional development goals, celebrating these successes reinforces the commitment to excellence.

3. IIDR Workshops and Webinars: The Indian Institute of Dental Research (IIDR) conducts workshops and webinars as part of a comprehensive 60-hour training module shot over two years. These educational sessions cover the latest advancements in dental care, best practices, and new technologies. By participating in these training programs, dental professionals stay at the forefront of their field, continuously enhancing their skills and knowledge.

Conclusion

Executing treatment with excellence is the culmination of the foundational pillars of dentistry. It involves a steadfast commitment to quality care, from the techniques used to the overall patient experience. By going above and beyond to ensure patient comfort and satisfaction, dental professionals can transform lives, bringing joy and relief to those they serve. Through advanced techniques, holistic approaches, continuous learning, and a culture of compassion, dental professionals make a positive difference in their patients' lives. As we continue to build on the pillars of exceptional care, the commitment to executing treatment with excellence remains at the heart of our practice, ensuring that every patient receives the highest standard of care tailored to their unique needs and journey.

Noting Progress Potential: Empower Patient Through Education

In the previous chapters, we explored the various pillars of dentistry, focusing on delivering exceptional care and ensuring patient satisfaction. Now, we turn to the sixth pillar of The Royal Ritual: Noting Progress Potential. This pillar emphasises the importance of empowering patients through education, enabling them to take charge of their oral health journey with newfound knowledge and confidence. Patient education is a cornerstone of effective dental care, leading to better treatment outcomes and long-term oral health.

Pillar 6: Noting Progress Potential: Empower Patient Through Education

Empowering patients through education is a cornerstone of achieving long-term oral health success. Dr. Arun Chamria's practice exemplifies this philosophy by prioritizing patient education, meticulous documentation, and open communication. This chapter explores the systematic approach taken to educate patients, highlighting follow-up protocols, innovative product development, and the essential role of detailed records in enhancing treatment outcomes. By understanding their oral health and the treatments available, patients can make informed decisions and take an active role in their care.

Third Generation Dental Clinic through Referrals

An astounding 95% of Dr. Chamria's patients continue their dental care with him for over 10 years. This long-term retention underscores the trust and satisfaction patients have in his services. Approximately 70% of new patients come through referrals from existing patients. This high referral rate highlights the positive experiences and successful outcomes that Dr. Chamria's patients share with others.

Documenting patient data and noting progress are cornerstones in the field of medicine, particularly in dentistry. Accurate data collection and meticulous record-keeping enable healthcare professionals to make informed decisions, predict outcomes, and tailor treatments to individual needs. This scientific approach is pivotal in advancing medical science and developing effective treatments.

From treating grandparents to parents and now their children, Royal Dental under Dr Chamria's guidance has come a long way. For older patients, the addition of a general anaesthesia machine has been a masterstroke in addressing dental anxiety. For parents with limited mouth opening or gag reflex issues, the implementation of intraoral scanning has significantly alleviated their concerns. For children, having an orthodontist on board with in-house aligner technology has made treatment more accessible and effective.

28+ Years Later: A Patient's Return for Dental Care

Recently, a remarkable instance underscored the value of meticulous documentation. A 90+ year-old patient visited Dr. Chamria's clinic for the first time in three decades. Initially, she believed this was her first visit. However, upon checking the clinic's records, it was revealed that she had received dental treatment from Dr. Chamria at the age of 60. This revelation not only amazed the patient but also highlighted the lasting impact of comprehensive record-keeping. The clinic had detailed records of her previous treatments as well as those of her family members. Now, three decades later, she returned for full-mouth restoration, underscoring the trust and continuity fostered through diligent documentation.

In Dr. Arun Chamria's practice, documenting patient progress is not just about keeping records; it's about empowering patients, enhancing treatment outcomes, and building lasting relationships. The success and loyalty of his patients are a testament to the profound impact of thorough documentation and patient-centered care. By continuously noting progress and refining treatments, Dr. Chamria sets a benchmark in the field of dentistry, demonstrating that meticulous attention to detail and patient education are key to long-term success and satisfaction.

Follow-Up Protocol: Ensuring Consistent Progress

Regular follow-ups are crucial in monitoring patient progress and ensuring the effectiveness of treatments. Dr. Chamria's practice emphasizes a structured follow-up schedule to keep patients engaged and informed:

1. 3 Days Post-Treatment: Initial check-up to assess immediate reactions and address any concerns.
2. 1 Week: Evaluation of healing progress and reinforcement of care instructions.
3. 1 Month: Comprehensive review of treatment effectiveness and adjustments as needed.
4. 3 Months: Ongoing assessment to ensure long-term stability and patient adherence to recommended practices.
5. 6 Months: Mid-term evaluation to monitor oral health maintenance and address any emerging issues.
6. 1 Year: Annual review to assess overall oral health and plan for future care needs.

Impact of Patient Education on Treatment Outcomes

Educating patients about their dental conditions and treatment options leads to better treatment outcomes and improved long-term oral health. When patients understand the rationale behind their treatment plans, they are more likely to comply with recommendations and take an active role in their care.

Educated patients are more likely to adopt preventive measures and maintain good oral hygiene practices, leading to long-term health benefits. Regular check-ups, cleanings, and early intervention for dental issues prevent the progression of diseases and reduce the risk of complications.

Simple yet essential tools like the case paper at Royal Dental offer comprehensive reporting on all teeth and treatment options, ranging from emergency care to preventive and rehabilitative procedures. The history paper is designed to capture detailed patient and family histories. During the initial consultation, intraoral scanning provides in-depth insights into each tooth. The consulting process is divided into two parts: taking medical history and addressing dental issues. In addition to the consultation, intraoral scanning and X-rays are also performed to ensure a thorough assessment.

Enhanced Compliance and Cooperation

Patient education fosters compliance and cooperation, which are crucial for successful treatment. For example, when patients understand the importance of maintaining oral hygiene after periodontal treatment, they are more likely to follow post-treatment care instructions, leading to better outcomes.

Dr. Chamria also established standard and customized prescriptions for patients undergoing various combinations of treatments. Under his guidance, Dr. Chirag Chamria developed an engaging Dental Assistant Training Workshop, which helps the team develop precise skills and master daily procedures. This comprehensive program ensures that all staff members are well-equipped to provide the highest level of care to patients, enhancing overall treatment outcomes and patient satisfaction.

Innovative Product Development: Enhances Oral Health

Dr. Chamria's commitment to patient well-being extends to the creation of proprietary oral care products. The development of natural and artificial toothpaste and mouthwash is a testament to this dedication. These products are formulated to cater to the diverse needs of patients, ensuring optimal oral hygiene and health.

Using Crown White toothpaste both in the morning and at night as part of your daily routine can significantly extend the lifespan of your dental crowns. Additionally, combining it with the recommended mouthwash helps reduce bacterial growth, treats gum disease, and maintains fresh breath for an extended period.

Build Trust and Rapport Through Open Communication

Effective patient education requires building trust and rapport through open communication. Dentists must create a comfortable environment where patients feel heard and valued. Here's how building trust and open communication can enhance patient education:

- **Listening to Patient Concerns**

Active listening is the foundation of effective communication. By listening to patients' concerns and addressing their fears, dentists can build trust and create a supportive environment. When patients feel understood, they are more likely to engage in open discussions about their health.

- **Provide Clear and Accessible Information**

Dentists should provide information in a clear and accessible manner. Avoiding technical jargon and using visual aids can help patients grasp complex concepts. For example, showing images of healthy gums versus gums affected by periodontal disease can make the information more relatable and understandable.

- **Encourage Questions and Discussions**

Encouraging patients to ask questions and participate in discussions about their treatment fosters a sense of partnership. Dentists should take the time to answer questions thoroughly and address any misconceptions. This interactive approach ensures that patients feel empowered and confident in their care.

- **Building Long-Term Relationships**

Open communication and trust-building lead to long-term relationships between patients and their dental care providers. When patients feel valued and supported, they are more likely to return for regular check-ups and follow through with treatment recommendations.

Celebrate Partnership Between Dentist and Patient

The partnership between dentists and patients is essential for achieving optimal oral health and well-being. This collaborative approach ensures that patients are active participants in their care, leading to better outcomes and increased satisfaction.

Education should be an ongoing process, not a one-time event. Providing patients with resources, such as brochures, videos, and online tools, can reinforce the information shared during visits. Regular follow-ups and check-ins also help to address any new concerns and provide additional support.

At our clinic, we offer an online portal where patients can access educational materials and track their oral health progress. This resource empowers patients to stay informed and engaged in their care between visits. Regular newsletters with tips and updates further support their journey to optimal oral health.

Best Practices for Scheduling Patient Appointment

At any Dental Clinic, one common obstacle is the variability in patient compliance and follow-up adherence. Patients may miss scheduled appointments or fail to follow prescribed care routines, leading to incomplete or inconsistent progress data. Additionally, maintaining accurate and comprehensive records can be challenging, especially when dealing with a high volume of patients or complex treatment plans. Inconsistent documentation practices among different staff members can also lead to discrepancies in patient records, affecting the overall quality of care.

This approach inspired the development of both physical and digital records, along with an online virtual calendar for managing the patient database. The team also created a custom CRM system and mobile app to streamline appointment scheduling and reminders. This online virtual suite has significantly alleviated labour-related issues, improving efficiency and accuracy in managing patient information.

First, implementation of a standardized documentation system ensured consistency across all patient records. This system includes detailed templates and checklists for recording patient histories, treatment plans, and follow-up notes. By adopting electronic health records (EHR), Royal Dental streamlines the documentation process, making it easier to update and access patient information in real-time.

Regular training sessions are conducted for staff members to ensure they are proficient in using the EHR system and adhere to best practices for documentation. Additionally, automated reminders and follow-up scheduling help ensure that patients adhere to their treatment plans and attend necessary appointments.

Role of Technology in Progress Tracking

When discrepancies or unexpected results occur, Royal Dental addresses them through a systematic review and resolution process. Discrepancies are identified via routine audits and quality checks of physical and digital records. If an issue arises, the practice promptly investigates by reviewing patient data and consulting with the healthcare team. The online virtual suite aids this process by offering centralized access to patient information, simplifying the identification and resolution of inconsistencies.

For example, if a patient reports missing an appointment, forgetting records, or needing details about treatment, billing, or referrals, the CRM system and mobile app at Royal Dental efficiently address these concerns. The CRM allows the team to verify appointments, retrieve records, and provide information on treatments, bills, and referrals. The mobile app ensures patients receive timely reminders and can easily access or update their information. This integrated system improves patient experience by delivering accurate, on-demand responses and reducing administrative burdens.

Conclusion

Empowering patients through education is a fundamental aspect of exceptional dental care. By providing knowledge, building trust, and fostering open communication, dentists can help patients take charge of their oral health journey. This empowerment leads to better treatment outcomes, long-term oral health, and a more positive overall experience.

As we continue to build on the pillars of dentistry, the commitment to patient education remains at the heart of our practice. By celebrating the partnership between dentists and patients, we can achieve optimal oral health and well-being for everyone we serve. This collaborative approach not only transforms smiles but also enhances the quality of life for our patients, creating a lasting impact that goes beyond the dental chair.

Tracking Follow-up & Summarizing: Ensuring Continuity of Care

In the previous chapters, we have explored the various pillars of dentistry that contribute to exceptional patient care. Now, we turn to the seventh and final pillar of The Royal Ritual: Tracking Follow-up & Summarizing. This pillar focuses on ensuring continuity of care through diligent follow-up, thorough documentation, and the fostering of lasting relationships between patients and their dental care team. Continuity of care is vital for maintaining and enhancing oral health, leading to patient satisfaction and loyalty.

Pillar 7: Tracking Follow-up & Summarizing: Ensuring Continuity of Care

Ensuring continuity of care means going beyond the initial treatment to provide ongoing support and attention. It involves regular follow-up visits, detailed documentation, and a commitment to building lasting relationships. This approach not only enhances patient outcomes but also creates a sense of trust and loyalty.

Dr. Chirag once recounted a memorable trip he took with his father, Dr. Arun, to Singapore in 2012 to attend the

International Dental Show (IDS). The conference was bustling with delegates from around the world, including exhibitors, visitors, speakers, and other attendees. During the event, Dr. Chirag was struck by the immense effort required to manage such a large-scale show. He remarked to his father on the extensive work involved, to which Dr. Arun responded with a notable comparison.

Dr. Arun explained that managing the IDS was not unlike their daily operations at Royal Dental. Just as the conference required meticulous coordination, their practice relies on a comprehensive appointment management approach. At Royal Dental, the process begins with calling patients to confirm their appointments and sending SMS reminders. They follow up with patients a day before their appointments and check on the day of the appointment to ensure timely arrival. This meticulous approach to appointment management and follow-up ensures a seamless experience for patients and helps maintain continuity of care.

Dr. Arun’s analogy highlighted the importance of a holistic appointment booking system in tracking and following up with patients effectively, paralleling the organization required for managing a major international event.

Sharing Anecdotes of Patients' Loyalty and Appreciation

Patients often demonstrate their loyalty and appreciation through their feedback on the personalized care and attention they receive during follow-up visits. One notable example is a patient who travelled from Zimbabwe to visit Dr Chamria back in 2008. This patient underwent a series of implants and dental crowns in a single day. The exceptional care he received—from the initial appointment booking over the phone to the final treatment and follow-up—left a lasting impression. He shared his positive experience with family and friends, highlighting the meticulous attention he received throughout his visit.

When this patient returned a few years later for a follow-up and to complete additional treatment, the staff at the reception made a memorable gesture. They reminded him of the famous Bombay Toast and tea he had ordered during his previous visit and offered to place a new order for him. The patient was both surprised and delighted by the staff's attention to detail and their recollection of his past experience. This thoughtful follow-up not only reinforced his loyalty but also exemplified the personalized care that defines Royal Dental's commitment to patient satisfaction.

Highlight Moments of Connection and Camaraderie

A memorable instance of connection and camaraderie occurred with a patient who travelled from the Middle East seeking deep scaling and advice on oral hygiene. During his visit, the patient first had a 30-minute consultation, followed by a more in-depth 45-minute session with Dr. Arun Chamria. Dr. Chamria's thorough and attentive approach addressed all of the patient's concerns, which led him to choose both oral prophylaxis and bite balancing on the same day.

The patient's satisfaction with the exceptional hospitality was so profound that he left a tip exceeding the cost of the treatment. When the staff inquired about the unusually generous tip, the patient responded, "Sometimes, how you make someone feel is more important than what you do for them." This poignant feedback highlighted not just the quality of the medical care provided but also the significant impact of making patients feel truly valued and cared for, reinforcing the importance of personal connection in delivering exceptional patient experiences.

Dental Treatment as a Precious Gift for Daughter

A busy morning at Royal Dental Clinics took an unexpected turn with a phone call from a concerned father. What made this call so remarkable? His daughter had struggled with crooked teeth from a young age, a concern that lingered despite her efforts to overlook it. Determined to give his daughter a new smile for her birthday, this father wanted to permanently address her dental issues and present her with a life-changing gift.

"The heart of a father is the masterpiece of nature."

Such gifts are rare—transformative and lasting, reshaping one's outlook on life. Back to the phone call: the father requested that the entire plan remain a secret. Upon the daughter's arrival at the clinic, she would be greeted with a series of surprises, including handwritten letters and well-wishes from friends and family, thoughtfully arranged in the consulting rooms. Every detail of this heartfelt plan was meticulously coordinated by the dedicated staff at Royal Dental Clinics. This is what patient follow-up and care stands for; it's magical in its own way. Dr. Arun Chamria laid the foundation for this belief: "One day of patience, many years of peace."

Thorough Documentation & Coordination

Thorough documentation and coordination are essential for providing seamless continuity of care. Accurate records ensure that every member of the dental team is informed and prepared to deliver consistent, high-quality care:

- **Role of Comprehensive Records:** Maintaining comprehensive records of each patient's treatment history, progress, and follow-up visits is crucial. These records enable dental professionals to monitor changes, track improvements, and make informed decisions about ongoing care. They also facilitate communication between different team members, ensuring that everyone is aligned in providing optimal care.
- **Coordination Among Dental Professionals:** Effective coordination among dental professionals enhances the quality of follow-up care. When dentists, hygienists, and assistants work together seamlessly, patients benefit from a cohesive approach to their oral health. This coordination is particularly important for complex cases that require multiple treatments and follow-up visits.

Celebrate Lasting Relationship Built on Trust and Respect

Lasting relationships between patients and their dental care team are built on trust and mutual respect. These relationships contribute to long-term oral health and patient satisfaction:

- **Trust Built Through Consistent Care:** Trust is earned through consistent, high-quality care and genuine concern for patients' well-being. When patients feel that their dental team is committed to their health and comfort, they are more likely to return for regular check-ups and follow-up visits.
- **Mutual Respect and Open Communication:** Mutual respect and open communication are key components of strong patient-dentist relationships. When patients feel respected and heard, they are more likely to engage in their care actively and follow through with treatment recommendations.

Impact of Personalized Follow-up Care

Personalized follow-up care is crucial, especially for patients who travel from afar or juggle busy work and home responsibilities. To accommodate their needs, it's essential to schedule appointments based on their convenience, and confirm these arrangements both verbally and through an online platform.

Consider the example of a patient who travels from a neighbouring city for regular check-ups. By offering flexible scheduling and confirming appointments through multiple channels, such as phone calls and text messages, the clinic ensures that the patient's time is respected and their travel is minimized.

A positive experience during follow-up visits goes beyond mere convenience; it enhances patient outcomes and builds long-term loyalty. For instance, a personalized approach might involve reminders tailored to the patient's specific treatment plan and regular check-ins to address any concerns they may have. This not only improves the overall patient experience but also fosters a sense of care and attentiveness that patients deeply appreciate.

Tailored Follow-up Plans

Creating tailored follow-up plans based on each patient's unique needs and circumstances ensures that they receive the most appropriate care. These plans consider factors such as the patient's medical history, treatment goals, and lifestyle.

Case Paper: This document includes detailed reporting on all teeth and potential treatments, covering emergency, preventive, and rehabilitative options. For example, we may want someone to help them understand the protocol at the reception itself or during first consultation.

History Paper: This paper involves gathering a detailed medical and family history of the patient, which is crucial for understanding their overall health and any potential impacts on dental care.

Intraoral Scanning: Performed during the first consultation, this provides detailed insights about each tooth, aiding in precise diagnosis and treatment planning. Maybe explaining the various tooth structures and treatments done to the patient will help build rapport.

Proactive Monitoring and Early Intervention

Proactive monitoring and early intervention are essential for preventing complications and ensuring the success of treatments. Regular follow-up visits enable dental professionals to identify potential issues before they become serious and to take timely, appropriate actions.

For instance, patients who were treated by Dr. Arun Chamria some years ago might return with new oral health concerns. In such cases, advanced diagnostic procedures—such as biopsies, zygomatic implants, or upgrading dental crowns—might be required. By addressing these evolving needs, we maintain a holistic approach to patient care, ensuring that each individual receives comprehensive and ongoing support.

This proactive approach not only enhances treatment outcomes but also demonstrates a commitment to the long-term health and well-being of our patients.

Strong Bonds and Lasting Loyalty

The strong bonds and lasting loyalty formed between patients and their dental care team are a testament to the importance of continuity of care. Continuity of care leads to transformative health improvements, as seen in patients who adhere to their follow-up plans and engage actively in their care. These improvements not only enhance oral health but also contribute to overall well-being.

Loyalty begins with the initial step of appointment booking, but Dr. Chirag's experience reveals how it truly manifests. Back in 2011, he observed his father managing a busy schedule, often seeing up to 30 patients a day. After each consultation, Dr. Arun would call a staff member into the room to reiterate the treatment plan, process, and payment details. This practice ensured clarity and consistency, fostering greater confidence and loyalty among patients.

This practice ensured that the staff was well-informed, the patient felt confident, and conversions were more likely. This attention to detail not only provided clarity but also fostered a deeper bond and trust between the patient and the clinic. Such moments of truth are crucial—they create a foundation of confidence and loyalty that strengthens the patient-clinic relationship.

Celebrating Follow-ups and Achievements

Celebrating milestones and achievements in patients' oral health journeys is crucial for emphasizing the importance of continuous care. Recognizing these accomplishments motivates patients to adhere to their treatment plans and fosters a sense of pride and satisfaction.

For instance, when the follow-up team successfully collects balance payments or facilitates treatment upgrades, their success is celebrated. If a team member converts a follow-up into a completed treatment or upgrade, the entire team is recognized, boosting morale and incentivizing individual efforts.

In addition to these recognitions, staff members are celebrated monthly, and birthdays and festivals are marked with special events. These celebrations build a sense of community and connection within the team. Recognizing achievements such as making calls, resolving queries, and following up on treatments highlights the collective effort that enhances patient care.

Weekly HR activities, like memory games, support staff development and communication skills, promoting professional growth and a positive work environment.

Conclusion

Tracking follow-up and summarizing is the culmination of the foundational pillars of dentistry. It involves ensuring continuity of care through diligent follow-up, thorough documentation, and the fostering of lasting relationships. By providing personalized attention and building strong connections, dental professionals can enhance patient outcomes, satisfaction, and loyalty.

As we continue to build on the pillars of exceptional care, the commitment to tracking follow-up and summarizing remains at the heart of our practice. Celebrating the success of continuity of care and the lasting relationships formed between patients and their dental care team underscores the importance of this pillar. It ensures that every patient receives the highest standard of care, tailored to their unique needs and journey, fostering a sense of trust, loyalty, and mutual respect.

Final Thoughts

As we reach the conclusion of this book, it's essential to reflect on the journey we have taken through the seven pillars of The Royal Ritual. It isn't easy to summarize what the pillars exemplify by way of excellence in the Indian dentistry. Each chapter has highlighted a critical aspect of dental care, emphasising the importance of a holistic, patient-centred approach. By integrating these pillars into daily practice, dental professionals can ensure they provide the highest standard of care, fostering long-term relationships with their patients and contributing to their overall well-being.

Success is not in Individualism, but in Professionalism

Dr. Chirag fondly recalls his time with his father, Dr. Arun Chamria, who was not only a skilled dentist but also the director of Royal Dental Clinics. "My father believed that I should handle administrative and lab duties," Dr. Chirag reminisces. "I used to wonder why a dentist would be tasked with such responsibilities. He made me sit at the reception, write prescriptions, and manage daily paperwork along with staff registers."

At the time, Dr. Chirag found these tasks perplexing. However, as he looks back, he realizes their immense value.

"Now I see the wisdom behind it," he reflects. "When a staff member is absent, I can allocate their work allocation seamlessly. I understand the processes thoroughly, ensuring systems are in place to prevent errors. Training and ongoing tasks have become simpler, allowing us to identify potential errors early and take corrective actions."

At Royal Dental Clinics, every dentist undergoes the same rigorous process. They start with a two-month induction at the reception, followed by a few weeks of assistance work, before beginning treatment duties. This comprehensive training ensures that each dentist is well-versed in all aspects of the clinic's operations, fostering a culture of excellence and meticulous care.

The Wisdom of a True Professional

Dr. Arun Chamria, the visionary behind Royal Dental Clinics, often shares a valuable lesson he learned from an inspirational mentor abroad. This lesson has become a cornerstone of the clinic's philosophy and training regimen. Dr. Arun once travelled to meet a renowned dentist who had a profound impact on his approach to the profession. During their conversations, the mentor shared a powerful piece of wisdom: "A professional is 33% academic knowledge, 33% economic management knowledge, and 33% knowledge of the prevailing laws."

Dr. Arun took this advice to heart and brought it back to Royal Dental Clinics. He understood that being an exceptional dentist required more than just clinical skills. It required a balanced combination of comprehensive knowledge.

He often recounted this wisdom to his team. "This is what I learned from that inspirational doctor abroad, and it's what I want to impart to all of you," he would say. He emphasized the importance of excelling in three key areas: academic excellence, economic management, and legal awareness.

Academic knowledge ensures that each dentist at Royal Dental Clinics stays at the forefront of dental science, providing patients with the best possible care based on the latest advancements.

Economic management knowledge enables the team to run the clinic efficiently, ensuring sustainability and growth. It also helps in making informed decisions about treatments and investments, ultimately benefiting the patients and the clinic.

Understanding prevailing laws is crucial for maintaining compliance with regulations and protecting the clinic and its patients. It fosters a sense of responsibility and ethics in all professional activities.

Dr. Arun's holistic approach to professional development has shaped the culture at Royal Dental Clinics. Each team member is encouraged to develop a well-rounded expertise, embodying the principles of comprehensive knowledge. This ensures that every patient receives not only top-notch clinical care but also benefits from a well-managed, legally compliant, and economically sound practice.

Through this story, Dr. Arun's legacy of balanced professionalism continues to inspire and guide the team at Royal Dental Clinics, setting a standard of excellence for years to come. This led to the foundation of The Royal Ritual and this book.

Overview of the 7 Steps of The Royal Ritual

1. Probing Patient Concerns: The Foundation of Exceptional Care
2. Analysing & Dismantling Problems: Precision in Diagnosis
3. Tracing Roots Causes: Unveil the Underlying Issues
4. Intuitive Treatment Planning: Crafting Personalized Solutions
5. Executing Treatment with Excellence: Prioritizing Quality Care
6. Noting Progress Potential: Empower Patient Through Education
7. Tracking Follow-up & Summarizing: Ensuring Continuity of Care

How to Implement These in Daily Routine

Implementing these seven steps of excellence into daily dental practice requires commitment, consistency, and a patient-focused mindset. Here's how dental professionals can integrate these pillars into their routine to achieve the best outcomes for their patients:

1. Probing Patient Concerns: The Foundation of Exceptional Care

- **Active Listening:** Dedicate time during each consultation to listen actively to your patients.

Encourage them to share their concerns, symptoms, and expectations without interruption.

- **Empathy and Understanding:** Approach each patient with empathy. Understand that their concerns might go beyond their immediate dental issues and consider their overall well-being.
- **Comprehensive History Taking:** Gather a detailed medical and dental history to identify any underlying conditions that may affect their oral health.

2. Analysing & Dismantling Problems: Precision in Diagnosis

- **Thorough Examinations:** Conduct comprehensive examinations, including visual inspections, palpations, and diagnostic tests such as X-rays and scans.
- **Detailed Documentation:** Keep meticulous records of all findings to track changes and ensure accurate diagnosis.
- **Collaborative Diagnosis:** Work with other dental specialists when necessary to ensure a comprehensive understanding of the patient's condition.

3. Tracing Root Causes: Unveiling the Underlying Issues

- **Holistic Approach:** Look beyond the symptoms to understand the root causes of dental issues. Consider factors such as diet, lifestyle, and systemic health conditions.

- **Patient Education:** Explain the underlying causes to patients in a way they can understand. This knowledge empowers them to take preventive measures.
- **Preventive Care Plans:** Develop preventive care plans tailored to address the root causes and prevent the recurrence of dental problems.

4. Intuitive Treatment Planning: Crafting Personalized Solutions

- **Customised Plans:** Develop treatment plans that are personalised to each patient's needs, preferences, and lifestyle.
- **Patient Involvement:** Involve patients in the decision-making process, explaining the benefits and risks of each treatment option.
- **Flexibility and Adaptation:** Be prepared to adjust treatment plans based on patient feedback and changing circumstances.

5. Executing Treatment with Excellence: Prioritizing Quality Care

- **Skill and Precision:** Maintain high standards of technical proficiency and stay updated with the latest advancements in dental techniques and technologies.

- **Patient Comfort:** Prioritize patient comfort during procedures. Use techniques such as sedation dentistry and pain management to ease anxiety.
- **Post-Treatment Care:** Provide detailed post-treatment instructions and follow-up to ensure proper healing and recovery.

6. Noting Progress Potential: Empowering Patients Through Education

- **Continuous Education:** Educate patients about their oral health, treatment options, and preventive care. Use visual aids and simple language to enhance understanding.
- **Engagement and Motivation:** Encourage patients to take an active role in their oral health by setting achievable goals and celebrating their progress.
- **Regular Communication:** Maintain open lines of communication to address any questions or concerns patients may have between visits.

7. Tracking Follow-up & Summarizing: Ensuring Continuity of Care

- **Consistent Follow-up:** Schedule regular follow-up visits to monitor progress and address any emerging issues.
- **Comprehensive Summarization:** Summarize each patient's treatment journey, including diagnoses, treatments, and outcomes, to provide a clear overview of their oral health.

- **Building Relationships:** Foster strong relationships with patients through consistent, personalised care and open communication.

A Ritual of Calm and Focus

One of the most endearing practices observed at Royal Dental Clinics is Dr. Arun Chamria's unique ritual before meeting each patient. "Every time we saw Dr. Arun enter a room, he would take something out of his pocket and use it," Dr. Chirag recalls. "Initially, we weren't sure what it was, but eventually, we mustered the courage to ask him."

Dr. Arun explained, "It's something that neutralizes me and centres my thoughts, so when I am with a patient, I am completely present. There are no intrusive thoughts overpowering my focus." This simple habit kept him calm and enabled him to give his best to each patient.

This practice of finding an object or ritual to ground oneself is a powerful lesson. For some, it's a prayer; for others, it's remembering loved ones or holding a special pen or instrument. For Dr. Arun, it was his ittar, a fragrant essence that symbolized calm and clarity.

In conclusion, the Royal Ritual pillar is more than a tradition; it's a testament to the dedication, meticulous training, and personal rituals that define the culture of Royal Dental Clinics. It's these practices that ensure every patient receives the highest level of care and every staff member embodies the clinic's commitment to excellence. The essence of success in dentistry lies not in individual accomplishments but in a collective commitment to professionalism.

Collaboration and Teamwork

- **Interdisciplinary Collaboration:** Work closely with other dental specialists, hygienists, and support staff to provide comprehensive care. Each team member's expertise contributes to the overall success of the practice.
- **Continuous Learning:** Engage in ongoing professional development to stay updated with the latest advancements in dental care. Attending conferences, participating in workshops such as IIDR, and pursuing further education.
- **Mentorship and Guidance:** Experienced professionals should mentor and guide newer practitioners, sharing knowledge and best practices to elevate the entire team.

Patient-Centered Approach

- o **Building Trust:** Establish trust with patients by consistently providing high-quality care and demonstrating genuine concern for their well-being.
- o **Open Communication:** Maintain transparency with patients about their treatment options, progress, and any potential risks. Clear communication fosters trust and ensures patients feel involved in their care.
- o **Personalised Care:** Treat each patient as an individual, tailoring treatments to their specific needs and preferences. Personalised care enhances patient satisfaction and outcomes.

Ethics and Integrity

- **Adherence to Ethical Standards:** Uphold the highest ethical standards in all aspects of practice, from patient interactions to business operations.
- **Transparency in Treatment:** Be honest and transparent with patients about their diagnoses, treatment options, and costs. Integrity builds trust and fosters long-term relationships.
- **Commitment to Excellence:** Strive for excellence in every aspect of dental care, continuously seeking ways to improve and innovate.

Community Involvement

- **Community Outreach:** Engage in community outreach programs to educate the public about oral health and provide services to underserved populations.
- **Patient Education:** Extend education beyond the clinic by providing resources, hosting workshops, and participating in public health initiatives.
- **Giving Back:** Contribute to the community by supporting local events, charities, and organisations that promote health and well-being. Royal Dental Clinics has reached out to about half a million citizens across Mumbai for oral health camps. Their intention is to serve those who serve the society.

Celebrating the Journey of Excellence

As we conclude this book, it's important to celebrate the journey of 40+ years of excellence in dentistry. The seven pillars we have explored provide a roadmap for dental professionals to deliver exceptional care and build lasting relationships with their patients. By embracing these principles and integrating them into daily practice, dental professionals can make a significant impact on their patients' lives and the broader community.

Wrap-Up

The journey to excellence in dentistry is ongoing, requiring dedication, compassion, and a commitment to continuous improvement. By embracing the seven pillars of excellence, dental professionals can provide exceptional care that transforms lives and fosters long-term relationships built on trust and mutual respect.

As you implement these principles in your daily practice, remember that success in dentistry is not achieved through individualism but through professionalism. It is the collective effort of a dedicated team, the commitment to ethical practice, and the focus on patient-centered care that drive true excellence. Celebrate the milestones, learn from the challenges, and continue striving for excellence in every aspect of your practice.

Thank you for joining us on this journey through the pillars of excellence in dentistry. We hope that the insights and strategies shared in this book will inspire and guide you in your quest to provide the highest standard of care for your patients, fostering a healthier, happier community.